THE
EVERYTHING.
GUIDE TO
LYME DISEASE

Dear Reader,

Since you picked up this book, I assume you may be curious or have a lot of questions about Lyme disease. I have been doing research on ticks and tick-borne diseases for over fifteen years. During this time, I have often been approached by people who wanted to learn more about my work. Some were fascinated that I work with ticks. Others asked about my insights into Lyme disease. Speaking to them, I realized that there is a wide range of views and misconceptions about Lyme disease, and tick-borne diseases in general. The topic of Lyme disease can be complex, and invokes a lot of passion in many people. I wrote this guide with the hope that it will assist you in understanding what Lyme disease is and clear up any misunderstandings you may have about this illness. What I wanted to provide you with is a book that has all of the current scientific facts about Lyme disease, but also one that describes alternative beliefs and the reasons people have them. I hope you find this book informative, interesting, and, most important, useful in helping you prevent this illness.

Dr. Rafal Tokarz

Welcome to the EVERYTHING® Series!

These handy, accessible books give you all you need to tackle a difficult project, gain a new hobby, or even brush up on something you learned back in school but have since forgotten. You can choose to read from cover to cover or just pick out information from our four useful boxes.

 Alerts

Urgent warnings

 Facts

Important snippets of information

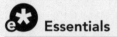 **Essentials**

Quick handy tips

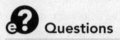 **Questions**

Answers to common questions

When you're done reading, you can finally
say you know **EVERYTHING**®!

PUBLISHER Karen Cooper

MANAGING EDITOR Lisa Laing

COPY CHIEF Casey Ebert

ASSOCIATE PRODUCTION EDITOR Jo-Anne Duhamel

ACQUISITIONS EDITOR Lisa Laing

DEVELOPMENT EDITOR Zander Hatch

EVERYTHING® SERIES COVER DESIGNER Erin Alexander

Visit the entire Everything® series at www.everything.com

THE
EVERYTHING
GUIDE TO
Lyme
Disease

From symptoms to treatments, all you need
to manage the physical and psychological
effects of Lyme disease

RAFAL TOKARZ, PhD

Adams Media

New York London Toronto Sydney New Delhi

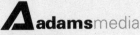

Adams Media
An Imprint of Simon & Schuster, Inc.
57 Littlefield Street
Avon, Massachusetts 02322

An Everything® Series Book.
Everything® and everything.com® are registered
trademarks of Simon & Schuster, Inc.

First Adams Media trade paperback edition May 2018

For information about special discounts for bulk purchases,
please contact Simon & Schuster Special Sales at 1-866-506-1949 or
business@simonandschuster.com.

The Simon & Schuster Speakers Bureau can bring authors to your live event. For
more information or to book an event contact the Simon & Schuster Speakers
Bureau at 1-866-248-3049 or visit our website at www.simonspeakers.com.

Manufactured in the United States of America

10 9 8 7 6 5 4 3 2 1

Library of Congress Cataloging-in-Publication Data has been applied for.

ISBN 978-1-4405-7709-3
ISBN 978-1-4405-7710-9 (ebook)

Acknowledgments

A special thank you to Esther, Aaron, Brian, Harvey, Iris, James, and Beata for their support. I could not have completed this book without your help. Jorge and Ian, thank you for the mentorship.

Contents

Introduction

Fifty years ago, there was no such thing as Lyme disease. The disease that we now call Lyme disease was a rare illness that had not yet been properly characterized. Since its discovery, Lyme disease has gone on to become one of the most frequently occurring infectious diseases in the United States. Current estimates indicate that approximately 300,000 Americans are diagnosed with Lyme disease each year, indicating a tremendous public health problem. It can be a difficult disease to face, filled with a wide variety of symptoms. In addition, many patients complain of persistent symptoms long after the disease is believed to be cured, which can have a profound effect on their lives.

Despite the vast amount of progress that has been made in learning about Lyme disease, there is still a great deal of mystery and confusion surrounding it. If you are reading this book, chances are you have either been personally affected by Lyme disease or you are worried about how it could affect you if you were to acquire it. Perhaps you have seen it in the news recently and are seeking explanations for why there seems to be so much controversy and misunderstanding about this disease.

If you search for answers about Lyme disease on the Internet, you can find many websites that will explain how it is transmitted and diagnosed, what the symptoms are, and what you can expect if you get infected. Some of what you find may even be accurate. Unfortunately, you will also find a great deal of misinformation. In fact, some people within the Lyme disease community can't agree on things such as what Lyme disease actually is, what the symptoms are, and how to treat it.

This book is a comprehensive resource for Lyme disease. It will familiarize you with all the different aspects of Lyme disease and provide you with the answers to a number of pressing questions that you may have about this illness. It will also help you sort through the different opinions about what this disease really is. By examining the history of Lyme disease, you will become aware of the factors that have led to the incredible expansion of this illness over the past few decades. This book will guide you through the various phases of the disease and the concerns regarding diagnosis and treatment. And, of course, you will learn a lot about ticks and how they contribute to the overall problem of not just Lyme disease, but other diseases as well. Just as important, you will also learn how to avoid ticks, and what to do if you are bitten. By the time you reach the end of this book, you will have a solid understanding of what this disease is and how to prevent it.

CHAPTER 1

What Is Lyme Disease?

If you have been diagnosed with Lyme disease, you are certainly not alone. In the United States, hundreds of thousands of people contract this disease every year. Even if you've never had it, you may have heard stories about how Lyme disease can be a severe and debilitating disease. Unfortunately, it can also be very misunderstood. Because of how common it is in some parts of the United States, an incomplete understanding of the symptoms, and confusion about how it is diagnosed, Lyme disease has become a controversial topic that has occasionally led to a lack of trust between patients, doctors, and the scientific community. To better understand this disease, it is important to know what Lyme disease is and what it isn't.

History and Expansion of Lyme Disease

Many people consider Lyme disease a relatively new disease. In some ways it is, and in some ways it isn't. A more appropriate term would be to call it an "emerging disease," one that has increased in frequency in recent years. It's new in that fifty years ago there was no such thing as Lyme disease because it hadn't yet been classified as a distinct disease. This does not mean that it didn't exist before then or that people hadn't been contracting the disease, because it did and they had. In fact, scientific journals published reports of an illness that was likely Lyme disease during the first half of the twentieth century, long before it was first characterized as a distinct disease. However, the first characterization of Lyme disease occurred just a little over forty years ago.

 Fact

> Lyme disease is known as an "infectious disease." Unlike diseases such as autoimmune diseases or most cancers that are usually caused by some sort of genetic abnormality, infectious diseases are caused directly by outside agents such as viruses, bacteria, or fungi, which are called "pathogens"—microbes that cause disease.

Discovery of Lyme Disease

The word "Lyme" in "Lyme disease" comes from the name of a town in Connecticut where the disease was first comprehensively studied. The very first detailed investigation of this disease started in November of 1975 when two mothers from the small town of Old Lyme, Connecticut, each independently alerted state and local health officials of a mysterious outbreak of arthritis in the town. One mother notified the state officials that twelve children out of the community of five thousand were diagnosed with a disease called juvenile rheumatoid arthritis.

Four of these children lived close together, on the same road. The second mother told the local health authorities that she, her husband, two of their children, and several of their neighbors all had arthritis as well. This alarmed the state health authorities because juvenile rheumatoid arthritis is random, meaning that many people coming down with the disease in so small a town was highly unusual. These alerts led to researchers setting up a surveillance program in Old Lyme, as well as in two surrounding towns—Lyme and East Haddam—in order to study this illness and possibly identify other people infected with the disease.

Between December of 1975 and May of 1976, a study led by doctors Allen Steere and Stephen Malawista identified fifty-one residents out of a total community population of twelve thousand that were affected with a similar illness, thirty-nine of whom were children. While talking to the patients, the doctors learned that all but one began to experience the symptoms after July 1972 and most often in the summer months. Their symptoms always began with sudden swelling and pain, usually in the knees.

❓ Question

What is juvenile rheumatoid arthritis?

Juvenile rheumatoid arthritis, also called juvenile idiopathic arthritis, is the most common cause of arthritis in children. It is an autoimmune disease, meaning the person's own immune system attacks some part of the body. The cause (or causes) is currently unknown.

Although the first attack usually went away within a week, the arthritis often came back several times after that, and many of the patients also reported having typical symptoms of the flu, such as fever, muscle pain, and general tiredness. About one quarter of the patients said they had an odd expanding rash. The center and outer edge were red, but the middle was clear, making it appear like a bull's-eye. This rash generally appeared about one month before the beginning of the arthritis. Interestingly, Drs. Steere and Malawista thought the description of the rash was similar to one first described in Europe in the early 1900s that was believed to be caused by tick bites. Both the physicians and the patients thought the rash was a result of an insect bite, but only one person recalled being bitten by a tick at the site of the rash.

This mysterious illness also appeared to have a particular geographic pattern. The area around these three towns was surrounded by woods, where deer, and the ticks that fed on them, were common. The patients experiencing this mysterious arthritic illness all lived near one another on large wooded lots or farms, where they presumably could come in contact with ticks. Of the thirty-nine affected children, seventeen lived on country roads.

In early 1977, the findings of the study were published and were the first to describe a new illness that was characterized by recurring attacks of arthritis. The illness was initially called "Lyme arthritis," before being slightly modified to Lyme disease. In a follow-up to their initial study, Drs. Steere and Malawista identified thirty-two new patients in the summer of 1976 who all appeared to suffer from "Lyme arthritis." This study helped define a lot of the symptoms we now associate with Lyme disease. Unlike the last study, this time most patients had a "bull's-eye" rash prior to symptoms, confirming that the appearance of the rash and the disease were linked. Three patients remembered being bitten by a tick at the site of the rash prior to its appearance, four patients had evidence of neurologic disease, and two more had problems with their heart, revealing that this illness was not limited to the skin and arthritis but affected other parts of the body as well. In addition, eight of the new patients came from outside of Connecticut, meaning the disease was found outside of the Lyme area. Within two years, a similar disease was reported in Wisconsin and as far away as the Pacific Coast and Europe.

By 1980, scientists learned that Lyme disease could be successfully treated with antibiotics, which then became the standard method of treatment. The actual cause of Lyme disease, and the fact that it was transmitted by ticks, remained a mystery until 1982, when it was finally identified by a group of scientists led by Dr. Willy Burgdorfer. As so often happens in science, it was identified by accident. Dr. Burgdorfer and his colleague Dr. Jorge Benach were studying a tick-borne disease called Rocky Mountain spotted fever. Although the pathogen causing this illness was known to be transmitted by ticks called American dog ticks, they wanted to see if other ticks could transmit this pathogen as well. The group collected blacklegged ticks (frequently also called deer ticks) on Shelter Island, New York, and used a microscope to analyze the microorganisms that lived inside the ticks.

Although they didn't find the agent of Rocky Mountain spotted fever, they found something else they thought was interesting. They discovered that more than half of the ticks contained unique, spiral-shaped bacteria. The scientists tested the blood of patients with Lyme disease and found that at some time in the past, they all had previously been infected with this bacteria. A year later, the same bacteria was found in the blood, cerebrospinal fluid, and skin of Lyme disease patients. These studies conclusively showed that this previously unknown bacteria, subsequently named *Borrelia burgdorferi* in Dr. Burgdorfer's honor, was indeed the cause of Lyme disease and that tick bites were the most likely way people were being infected.

e✱ Essential

Growing bacteria in a laboratory does not mean increasing its size. It means creating an environment where the bacteria are able to continuously divide on their own, away from their host.

Along with the discovery of the bacteria by Dr. Burgdorfer, another major breakthrough in studies of Lyme disease also occurred in 1982, when scientists led by Dr. Alan Barbour grew cultures of the bacteria in a laboratory for the first time. Although the bacteria was difficult to grow at first, scientists were able to figure out the right mix of different nutrients that allowed it to grow on its own. By identifying a method for studying *Borrelia burgdorferi* away from ticks or animal hosts, scientists all over the world could now study this bacteria like never before.

Early Cases of Lyme Disease

Contrary to its name, Lyme disease did not originate in Lyme. Lyme and the adjoining towns just happened to be where the disease was first recognized. By the time Drs. Steere and Malawista began their study in 1975, the disease had been occurring in many different regions of the United States but was not being recognized as a distinct illness. After its discovery by Drs. Steere and Malawista, it became clear that Lyme disease was not a new disease at all but went back nearly one hundred years prior to its discovery. In the early twentieth century there were many cases of this illness reported by doctors examining patients in Europe, although at the time it was obviously not yet known to be Lyme disease.

The first instance of someone with what was likely Lyme disease can be traced all the way back to 1883 in Germany, and doctors first learned of the rash (and its connection to tick bites) in 1909 in Sweden. This led to the rash being reported by physicians throughout Europe, usually linked to some bite of a blood-sucking pest such as a tick. One strange difference is that there was never any mention of arthritis in these European cases. This was likely due to how Lyme disease manifests in Europe—the course of the disease can be quite different following the initial rash, and arthritis is relatively rare. Even in the United States, there were reports of patients with a similar rash in Wisconsin and elsewhere in Connecticut in the early 1970s, just prior to the initial Lyme study, without a link to arthritis. Linking the rash and all of the different ways Lyme disease can manifest gave this disease a distinct identity that doctors could better diagnose and treat.

 Fact

Until *Borrelia burgdorferi* was clearly shown to be the cause of Lyme disease, there were many suggested causes of the rash, including tick-transmitted toxins, viruses, and other bacteria.

The Rise in Lyme Disease

At first, reports of Lyme disease were confined to a few states in the Northeast and around the Great Lakes, with just a few sporadic cases reported on the West Coast. As the 1980s progressed, the number of cases, and the number of states reporting them, began to grow. In 1982, the CDC began to informally track the disease, and finally, in 1991, Lyme disease became a nationally notifiable disease. This meant that each case was now required to be reported by the physician to the local health department, which would in turn be required to report it up the chain until the data was registered by the CDC. This allowed the CDC to keep better track of the number of cases each year, and by the mid-2000s, there were nearly 25,000 cases reported annually. Lyme disease was being reported all along the East Coast, from Maine down to Florida. It was also expanding west, with most states east of the Rocky Mountains now reporting the disease as well. Doctors in counties that had previously been thought to be free of Lyme disease were now seeing cases, and each year the numbers grew. Between 1993 and 2012, the number of counties with a high frequency of Lyme disease increased threefold, from 65 to 260. In the northeastern part of the country, Lyme disease became a major epidemic, with some states reporting up to 5,000 cases every year. In all, between 1982 and 2012, more than 350,000 cases of Lyme disease were reported by the CDC.

✪ Essential

The Centers for Disease Control and Prevention (CDC) is the main national health institute in the United States. The agency's main purpose is to protect public health through controlling and preventing diseases. The CDC tracks trends in infectious diseases and establishes guidelines for diagnosis and treatment.

As of 2017, Lyme disease was the seventh highest reportable disease in the United States. Anyone who gets bitten by the tick that carries *Borrelia burgdorferi* is at risk for Lyme disease. However, Lyme disease is most often diagnosed in children between the ages of five and fifteen and adults between the ages of forty-five and fifty-five. It is also slightly more common in men than women. In states where Lyme disease is common, children tend to be diagnosed more often, whereas in states where Lyme disease is less common, adults make up the majority of cases. Scientists are still not sure what causes this discrepancy or even if it's real; it could be that adults in non-endemic states are simply misdiagnosed.

 Fact

Reportable diseases are diseases where the CDC requires doctors to tell them about all cases they diagnose so they can track statistics and outbreaks. These are generally diseases where information is needed to help control the disease, such as measles, as opposed to common infectious diseases such as the cold or the flu.

The Cause of Lyme Disease Expansion

As we just learned, the disease that we now call Lyme disease has been here for a long time. So why did it emerge only in the past forty years? And why is it so common now? Although there probably is not a single answer to these questions, there are several possible reasons this disease has grown so much so quickly. The main reason most likely has to do with the geographic expansion of the ticks that transmit the disease. Ticks that transmit Lyme disease are more abundant than ever and can now be found in areas where they wouldn't have been half a century ago. This expansion has been driven by a variety of human and environmental factors, some of which will be examined in Chapter 2.

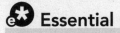 **Essential**

The term "endemic" is used to describe something that is frequent. A state such as Connecticut, where high numbers of Lyme disease are diagnosed each year, would be referred to as a Lyme disease–endemic state, whereas Colorado might be considered a non-endemic state.

There has also been more attention paid to Lyme and other tick-borne diseases in recent years, particularly in regions where ticks are common. With more information about Lyme disease available to the public, people are more likely to recognize signs of this illness and seek a Lyme disease diagnosis and treatment.

Lyme Disease Reporting

Almost from the beginning, there was a widespread belief among patients and clinical doctors that Lyme disease cases were significantly underreported. Many people were convinced that the annual number of Lyme disease cases that was listed by the CDC represented just a small portion of the actual number of people who came down with the disease. Studies performed in the 1990s looked at the reporting of Lyme disease in specific states and showed that Lyme disease was underreported by anywhere from one third to one twelfth the correct amount. More recent studies revealed that underreporting on a national level is just as high. Although the average number of reported annual cases now stands at around thirty to thirty-five thousand, recent studies by the CDC show that the true number of cases in the United States is likely ten times higher.

How did the CDC finally realize the true extent of annual cases of Lyme disease, especially since only a fraction is actually reported? First, they looked at the numbers of Lyme disease tests performed by large commercial laboratories in the United States and determined how many, on average, were positive. Then they analyzed the nationwide number of health insurance claims for patients with a diagnosis of Lyme disease. Both studies produced similar results and showed that more than 300,000 cases of Lyme disease occur in the United States each year.

There are many reasons such a huge discrepancy exists between the number of cases of Lyme disease that are reported and the number of actual cases that occur, such as failure by physicians to report the diagnosis, incomplete or missing case reports, and failure to pass the report from one health department to the next. Whatever the reasons, one thing is certain: Lyme disease is much more prevalent than previously thought.

Borrelia burgdorferi: The Lyme Disease Bacteria

Borrelia burgdorferi (abbreviated to *B. burgdorferi*) is the official scientific name of the bacteria that causes almost every case of Lyme disease in the United States. It is a type of bacteria known as a spirochete, meaning it is spiral shaped, like a tiny corkscrew. Spirochetes are long and very thin and look like a strand of very curly hair. They can live in a wide variety of different environments, and *Borrelia* are not the only spirochetes that people come in contact with. There are several other spirochetes that can cause human disease. For example, the bacteria that cause syphilis and leptospirosis are also spirochetes and in fact look identical to *B. burgdorferi*. There are also many spirochetes that live in us that do not cause disease—some even live in our mouths.

Where is *B. burgdorferi* found?

Unlike the various types of "common" bacteria that live in the environment all around you, *B. burgdorferi* needs to live inside another host at all times—either a tick, an animal, or a human.

This bacteria cannot survive in the outside environment, meaning *B. burgdorferi* cannot live on the floor, on your table, on your porch, or even in the soil in your backyard You cannot acquire it by touching an inanimate object, and it is not contagious, meaning it cannot be transmitted through direct contact with another person nor through the air, like the virus that causes the flu. If you are with someone with Lyme disease, you cannot get it by shaking the person's hand, by hugging, or by kissing. A cough or sneeze from an infected person is not infectious. Although some people claim that it can be sexually transmitted, there is no evidence indicating that it can be transmitted in such a manner. Although it is theoretically possible to acquire it through a blood transfusion (if the transfused blood was infected), this is very unlikely because of thorough blood testing. The only way *B. burgdorferi* can infect you is through the bite of an infected tick. Because the tick is a prerequisite to any disease transmission and *B. burgdorferi* are only present *inside* the tick, never on the outside, just having a tick crawling on your body will not lead to Lyme disease. If you see a tick crawling on your clothes or skin, just getting rid of it will prevent Lyme disease or any other tick-borne disease.

✅ Fact

Despite Dr. Burgdorfer being recognized as the first scientist to identify the spirochete that causes Lyme disease, a German scientist named Carl Lennhoff claimed in 1948 to observe spirochetes in the skin of patients with rashes similar to those sometimes seen in patients with Lyme disease.

Movement of *B. burgdorferi*

The ability to move varies among different bacteria. For example, the bacteria that cause staph infections or strep throat cannot move at all. However, there is one thing that spirochetes are very good at—they can move very quickly. *B. burgdorferi* is extremely mobile, a feature important in its ability to spread quickly during infection. In fact, this capability for quick movement is one of the most important factors in its ability to cause disease.

Unlike many pathogenic bacteria, *B. burgdorferi* does not directly infect the cells in your body. Instead, it is what is called an "extracellular bacteria," meaning it stays outside of your cells at all times. During infection, it uses its mobility to continuously move through your body. The bacteria basically "drills" through your skin and other tissues in order to move and infect other sites in your body. It does so not by moving through cells, but rather through spaces found in between cells. These spaces are called extracellular spaces, which is why *B. burgdorferi* is referred to as an extracellular bacterium.

❓ Question

Are the flagella found in animals and bacteria the same?
Both flagella perform the same function: they allow the cells to move. The methods of flagellar movement are different in animals and bacteria. In bacteria, the flagella move in a circular fashion, very much like a propeller. In animals, the flagella move in a wave-like manner.

B. burgdorferi can move so rapidly because it contains multiple flagella, which are long threadlike extensions that cells use for movement. Flagella are not unique to bacteria. For example, human sperm cells can "swim" because they have a flagellum that they use for movement. All spirochetes, *B. burgdorferi* included, have seven to eleven flagella. Interestingly, the front of each flagellum is attached at one end of the bacteria, then it's wrapped several times around the length of the bacteria, and the end is attached at the other end of the bacteria. When the bacteria moves, it rotates the flagella at one end. Because the flagella are wrapped around the bacteria, the entire bacteria rotates or twists as well. Think of it as holding a rope at each end and then twisting it on one end—the whole length of the rope eventually becomes twisted. This is why spirochetes are "spiral"; their cells continuously twist as they move. In fact, defective spirochetes that cannot make flagella are not spiral at all, but look like long, straight, thin threads.

Other Lyme Disease Bacteria

In the United States, more than ten different bacteria related to *B. burgdorferi* have been found in ticks, but until recently, only infection with *B. burgdorferi* was shown to cause disease. This changed in 2016, when a new bacteria, called *Borrelia mayonii*, was discovered at the Mayo Clinic in Minnesota and was also shown to cause Lyme disease.

ⓔ✔ Fact

In addition to *B. burgdorferi*, over fifty other bacteria can be found throughout the world that are also classified as *Borrelia*. These bacteria are all genetically and physiologically closely related to *B. burgdorferi*, but at the same time different enough to be given a different species name.

This distinct *Borrelia* bacteria was discovered almost by accident during routine blood testing for Lyme disease. Between 2012 and 2014, over ten thousand patient samples were tested for *B. burgdorferi* at the Mayo Clinic. Of the roughly one hundred samples that tested positive for *B. burgdorferi*, six appeared to have a different but related bacteria. After scientists investigated these bacteria further, it was conclusively proven that this was indeed a new species of *Borrelia*. The new bacteria was then given the scientific name *Borrelia mayonii* in honor of the institute where it was discovered. So far, only a few cases of Lyme disease due to this new bacteria have been reported, all in the upper Midwest (Minnesota,

North Dakota, and Wisconsin), and *B. burgdorferi* remains the main cause of Lyme disease in the United States.

Outside of the United States, however, the situation is quite different. In Europe, there are three main species that cause Lyme disease. One of them is *B. burgdorferi.* The other two are called *Borrelia garinii* and *Borrelia afzelii,* and in many areas in Europe, these two species are more common than *B. burgdorferi.* Interestingly, each species causes slightly different symptoms, although they all can cause a similar rash. Lyme disease caused by *B. garinii* and *B. afzelii* is also found throughout northern Asia and in Japan.

⊘ Fact

By comparing the genetic material of *B. burgdorferi* from the United States and from Europe, scientists determined that *B. burgdorferi* originated in Europe but has been present in North America for millions of years.

B. burgdorferi in Ticks and Animals

B. burgdorferi can live in ticks and vertebrate animals, which are two very different hosts and very different environments for the bacteria to live in. You can think of it as alternating between living in the tropics and Antarctica. In order to do so, you would have to learn to adapt very quickly in order to face very different challenges. It works the same way with bacteria; scientists studying *B. burgdorferi* have learned that the bacteria changes drastically as it moves from the tick to an animal or vice versa.

When *B. burgdorferi* is in a tick, it is present in very low amounts, between about several hundred to several thousand bacteria. There are very few nutrients for the bacteria to live on and they do not divide or often move—they just sort of exist, using a protein called outer-surface protein A (OspA) to attach to the digestive system of the tick, called the tick gut. As the tick feeds, the incoming blood changes the gut of the tick from a nutrient-deprived environment to one that is highly nutritious. The blood signals to *B. burgdorferi* that it's going to enter a new environment, which "awakens" the bacteria.

 Fact

> The tick gut is different from a stomach as you might imagine it. An animal's stomach digests food before it goes to the intestines to absorb nutrients. The tick gut both digests the food and absorbs the nutrients in the same organ.

At that point, *B. burgdorferi* transforms. It becomes very active and begins to divide very quickly. It gets rid of OspA from its surface, detaches from the tick's gut, and sends up a wide variety of new proteins to the surface that it will need to enter and establish an infection in the new host. It drills through the tick's gut and then spreads throughout the body of the tick. Some of the bacteria wind up in the tick's salivary glands, from where they can be transmitted into another host. During feeding, the tick continuously injects saliva into the wound, and once the bacteria make it into the salivary gland, they too are injected into the new host along with the saliva. This ends the tick part of the *B. burgdorferi* life cycle and begins the human (or animal) infection, which presents a greater number of challenges for the bacteria, the most important of which is evading the immune system of the new host.

Fact

Along with the nutrients in the blood, temperature plays an important role in transforming *B. burgdorferi* from the "tick-infecting" type to the "human-infecting" type. The inside of the tick is typically at room temperature and is not the preferred temperature for the bacteria. During feeding, the incoming warm blood increases the temperature of the tick gut to body temperature. This is the preferred temperature for *B. burgdorferi* at which it divides more rapidly, moves more quickly, and can make the proteins that are necessary for animal infection.

The Battle with the Immune System

As soon as any foreign microbe enters your body, it is immediately attacked by your immune system. The vast majority of microbes are destroyed on the spot and will not cause disease, and you never even knew that you were infected. The pathogenic microbes must be able to overcome the initial response of your immune system and stay around long enough for you to eventually feel some kind of illness from the infection.

There are a number of ways that *B. burgdorferi* try to overcome your immune system. One way is through a process called "antigenic variation." This term refers to the bacteria continuously changing how it looks to fool the immune system. The way your immune system recognizes a pathogen is by first identifying unique proteins that are present on the surface of the pathogen and then destroying any organism that has that protein on its surface. Because your own cells won't have these proteins, they will not be affected. Early on during the infection, *B. burgdorferi* switches the proteins that it has on the surface and begins using other proteins. For example, a protein called outer-surface protein C (OspC), which is important for the bacteria early on in the infection, disappears from the surface of the bacteria. If your immune system searches for any bacteria with OspC, it won't find it. Among new proteins that the bacteria makes is a protein called VlsE (Variable Lipoprotein Surface-Exposed). VlsE is unique because *B. burgdorferi* can continuously change its shape to fool your immune system; in fact, it could theoretically make millions of different versions of VlsE. Each time your immune system learns how to eliminate one version, *B. burgdorferi* gets rid of it and makes a new one. And this process continues on and on. Your immune system eventually catches up, even without treatment, but it can take months or perhaps years until it does so.

Another way *B. burgdorferi* evades the immune system is by turning some of its parts off. Since it would not be good for the immune system to be turned on all the time, there are various proteins in our body that turn it off. As *B. burgdorferi* moves through the body, it sticks to some of these proteins, which causes parts of the immune system to turn off and thus be unable to destroy the bacteria. This is also where the ability for rapid movement is very helpful for *B. burgdorferi*. While some parts of our immune system that aren't turned off are trying to locate and destroy the bacteria, it can simply outrun them.

Alert

Many people use the term "infection" interchangeably with the term "disease." Though very often the two go hand in hand, sometimes they don't. An infection occurs when a microorganism first enters your body, while a disease occurs when the infection leads to some kind of damage in your body. Not all infections, even with pathogenic organisms, will cause disease.

Not All *B. burgdorferi* Are Created Equal

In order to learn more about *B. burgdorferi*, scientists analyze the genetic features of this bacteria. It turns out that there are many different types of *B. burgdorferi* in ticks throughout the continent.

Each type is slightly different from the others, with these small genetic differences affecting the extent of the disease when it infects a host. We call these slightly different types "strains." For example, we all have billions of harmless *E. coli* bacteria in our intestines. However, you can get sick by eating beef that has strains of *E. coli* from cattle, which are different from ours.

Some strains of *B. burgdorferi* can be carried by ticks but are not found in any humans or animals, meaning that, for whatever reason, they likely cannot cause disease in people. Other strains can be found in ticks but only in the skin of Lyme disease patients without it spreading to other areas of the body. These strains can cause some minor skin infections around the site of the bite, but never a more serious infection. Finally, there are strains that cause severe disease. These strains of *B. burgdorferi* travel much more easily from the tick bite to other parts of your body, meaning the infections spread more quickly. The strains of *B. burgdorferi* are each very different and which one you get will drastically affect the severity of your illness. It is not clear what exactly allows one strain to cause a more severe disease than another. However, the ability of some strains to evade the immune response better than others is likely a very important factor.

The Genome of *B. burgdorferi*

The first strain of *B. burgdorferi* that was isolated by scientists back in 1982 was called the B31 strain and came from ticks originating from Shelter Island, New York. Since this initial isolation, there have been hundreds, possibly thousands, of different *B. burgdorferi* strains isolated on different continents, but the B31 strain has probably been used in more scientific studies than any other. In 1997, in what was a huge scientific achievement, the *B. burgdorferi* B31 strain became the third bacteria that had its genome sequenced. This means its entire genomic material, or DNA, was identified. By identifying all of the *B. burgdorferi* genes, scientists could now study the bacteria on a genetic level. Because of this research, scientists could determine which *B. burgdorferi* genes are important for disease or which can potentially be used as future vaccine candidates.

 Fact

The B31 strain got its name from the three scientists involved in its isolation: Drs. Burgdorfer, Barbour, and Benach (the three Bs). The "1" denotes that it was the very first *B. burgdorferi* isolated away from a host. Hence, B31 stands for the three Bs, first isolate. This strain can cause severe disease.

How Exactly Does *B. burgdorferi* Cause Disease?

Having the ability to examine the genome of *B. burgdorferi* made it easier for scientists to try to identify different parts of this bacteria that could be responsible for the symptoms of Lyme disease. Many bacteria that cause human disease produce substances called extracellular toxins, which, when released from bacteria, have some harmful effects. Examining the genome, scientists learned that *B. burgdorferi* did not appear to produce any such toxins. Instead, it turned out that the main culprits of Lyme disease appear to be lipoproteins, a type of protein that *B. burgdorferi* has in abundance. It can produce over fifty different types of these proteins, many of which are called OSPs. It turns out that lipoproteins are incredibly effective at activating the human immune system, which results in high inflammation. Although inflammation is the standard way your immune system deals with pathogens, high inflammation unfortunately also results in damage to your own body. And this is in essence what a *B. burgdorferi* infection does to your body. Basically, Lyme disease is caused by inflammation in response to the presence of lipoproteins of *B. burgdorferi*.

Summary

With published reports of Lyme disease that go back to the nineteenth century, Lyme disease is definitely not a "new" disease. It got its name from an area in Connecticut where it was first identified as a distinct illness in the mid-1970s. It was initially diagnosed in a small cluster of people suffering from arthritis. Since then, Lyme disease has undergone a tremendous expansion in the United States, and according to the most recent estimates from the CDC, approximately 300,000 cases of this disease occur each year. It has become a global problem as well, with thousands of Lyme disease cases reported in Europe and Asia every year.

Lyme disease is caused by a spirochete bacteria called *B. burgdorferi* that is transmitted by tick bites. Although *B. burgdorferi* is unable to survive outside of a host, it has developed extraordinary survival mechanisms that allow it to live inside two very different types of hosts: ticks and warm-blooded animals such as humans.

This bacteria also has several components that make it a very problematic pathogen. It is highly mobile and it uses this ability to quickly move through the body during infection. It has an abundance of lipoproteins, which cause a high degree of inflammation that ultimately results in the symptoms of Lyme disease. On a genetic level, it is highly variable and has many ways to fool the immune system. All of these factors make *B. burgdorferi* very difficult to get rid of and contribute to the reasons Lyme disease is such a substantial problem.

CHAPTER 2

Transmission and Prevention

There are dozens of types of ticks around the United States and even more in the rest of the world. However, only a few of them can transmit *B. burgdorferi*. A better understanding of what they are and where and when they are active can help you avoid getting Lyme disease. This chapter will provide you with all the information you need to know about ticks, the crucial role they play in Lyme disease, and how to protect yourself from them.

All about the Tick

Ticks belong to a large group of animals called arthropods. This group includes insects, crustaceans, spiders, and any other invertebrates with segmented bodies, jointed limbs, and exoskeletons. Although most people think that ticks are insects, they are not. Ticks are arachnids like spiders, scorpions, or mites. There are many scientific differences between arachnids and insects, but the easiest way to tell them apart is by the number of legs present on each. Ticks and other arachnids have eight legs, whereas insects have only six.

Ticks, like mosquitoes, fleas, or lice, acquire all their nutrients by feeding on the blood of some other host, such as an animal or human. The two types of ticks you may encounter are hard ticks and soft ticks. The main difference is self-explanatory—hard ticks have a tough outer shell and are extremely difficult to crush (soft ticks, not so much). There are several other differences between hard and soft ticks. Soft ticks are generally found in caves, animal burrows, and simple human dwellings such as huts, cabins, or sheds, whereas hard ticks can frequently be found in the woods. Soft ticks typically feed at night, while hard ticks prefer the daytime. Soft ticks feed more frequently than hard ticks. They tend to feed quickly, detach, and come back for another meal. Hard ticks can feed for days, sometimes for up to two weeks. Soft ticks also can also live much longer than hard ticks; some are known to survive for up to sixteen years.

 Fact

Animals such as ticks, fleas, and mosquitoes are what we call "ectoparasites." A parasite is an organism that lives in or on another host and benefits from it, while causing the host harm. "Ecto" means outside; hence, ticks are parasites found outside the host's body.

The Blacklegged Tick

There are about ninety different species of ticks found in the United States. Of those ninety, only seven bite people frequently and a few others bite people on rare occasions. There are only two types of ticks that can carry and transmit *B. burgdorferi*, the bacteria that causes Lyme disease. The most common tick for transmitting Lyme disease, responsible for over 95 percent of all cases in the United States, is commonly known as the "blacklegged tick" or the "deer tick." The scientific name for this tick is *Ixodes scapularis*, usually abbreviated to *I. scapularis*. This tick is found throughout the eastern half of the United States. On the West Coast, Lyme disease is caused by bites of a very similar tick, commonly called the "western blacklegged tick" or *Ixodes pacificus* (abbreviated to *I. pacificus*) in scientific circles.

Both the blacklegged tick and its western counterpart are hard ticks. All hard ticks have three life stages: the larva, nymph, and adult. At each stage, they feed only once. This means that hard ticks feed three times in their entire life, which for blacklegged ticks is about two years. Each feeding provides the tick the necessary nutrients to move to the next stage of its life. The differences in life stages and the seasons at which they occur determine the likelihood of acquiring Lyme disease.

Larval Stage

Larval ticks hatch from eggs and feed between mid-August and September each year. They are incredibly small, about the size of the period at the end of this sentence. This makes them virtually impossible to notice. Fortunately, larval ticks cannot inherit *B. burgdorferi* from their parent ticks, so when they hatch in the summer, they are not infected and their bites do not cause Lyme disease. When they come out to feed, they are usually found in piles of leaves. Larval ticks typically find small animals to feed on, usually field mice, who are often infected with *B. burgdorferi*. When a larval tick feeds on an infected mouse, usually for about three days, it too acquires *B. burgdorferi* by feeding on the mouse's blood. Twenty-four hours after attachment, *B. burgdorferi* has most likely been transmitted into the larval tick. The bacteria can be found in large amounts within the tick after just forty-eight hours, even before it has drunk most of the blood, which usually occurs on the last day of feeding. Once the bacteria are inside, they establish a lifelong infection in the tick. Following the meal from its host, the larva drops off and spends the next six months or so hiding in vegetation. Around April, the larva will begin to molt and move on to the next life stage. It sheds its outer coating, grows in size, and becomes a nymph, the most important life stage for the transmission of Lyme disease.

Nymphal Stage

When nymphal ticks first arrive, many of them are already infected with *B. burgdorferi* and now can infect animals or people. Like larvae, nymphs are also typically found in piles of leaves or at the edge of wooded areas, beginning in the middle of May and staying through August. They come out as the weather grows warmer, when people go hiking or camping and kids spend much more time playing outside because schools are out for summer. All of these activities bring kids and adults in closer proximity to ticks.

Despite being twice the size of the larvae, nymphs are also still very small, approximately the size of a poppy seed, and extremely difficult to spot. The tiny size of nymphal ticks and the early summer feeding season are the two major reasons most Lyme disease cases come at the time of the year when the nymphs are active. Over 90 percent of Lyme disease cases in the United States are diagnosed at that time, with the peak in June and July.

Nymphs feed for three to four days. After a nymph feeds on a host (usually a mouse, just like the larvae), they molt to the final stage—the adult.

Adult Stage

At this stage, the tick can become either a male or female. Only females feed at this stage as they need a blood meal to produce eggs. Because males cannot feed, they do not transmit *B. burgdorferi*. The females have a characteristic orange-red abdomen and are two to three times larger than nymphs, making them easier to spot.

🅴❗ Alert

Although most photos of blacklegged ticks tend to show the large red female adults, it is the smaller darkish nymphs that are the main transmitters of Lyme disease.

Adults come out in the fall, typically in early October, and remain active throughout the winter until mid-spring if the temperature is high enough. Ticks are not active during cold winter days, but when the temperature climbs to over 45°F, adults can emerge and will bite. However, since adults are around at a time when people are less likely to be outside and adult ticks are easier to notice, adults make up only about 10 percent of all Lyme disease cases. Most female ticks end up feeding on large animals, frequently deer (where the name "deer tick" comes from), for five to seven days. After the female has fed, it will wait out the winter until laying eggs the following spring in May. A typical adult blacklegged tick female will lay about 1,000 to 3,000 eggs in one large mass. When the larvae hatch, the cycle then begins again.

Western Blacklegged Ticks

The western blacklegged tick has a slightly different life cycle than the blacklegged tick in the East, which makes it less likely to infect people with *B. burgdorferi*. During their nymphal and larval stages, the western blacklegged ticks prefer to feed on a lizard called the western fence lizard, which does not get infected with *B. burgdorferi*. Because the lizards don't become infected, they can't pass the *B. burgdorferi* infection on to other western blacklegged ticks that feed on them later. In addition, because most of the larval and nymphal ticks feed on these lizards, by the time these ticks become adults, very few are infected with *B. burgdorferi*—only roughly 1 percent. The ticks that are infected typically feed on different species of rats, which are the most frequent source of infection with *B. burgdorferi* for the western blacklegged ticks. This major difference in hosts by larval and nymphal ticks is the primary reason why the western blacklegged ticks are responsible for less than 5 percent of Lyme disease cases in the United States. In addition, due to the differences in climate between the coasts, the time of the year that the western blacklegged ticks come out to feed is also a bit different than for the blacklegged ticks. For example, the nymphs appear in mid-March and seek hosts until July.

ⓔ✓ Fact

Like the adult blacklegged tick females, adult western blacklegged tick females also usually feed on deer. The deer they feed on, called the Columbian black-tailed deer, is the primary type of deer present on the West Coast. The males do not feed.

Differentiating Blacklegged Ticks from Other Ticks

In many areas, blacklegged ticks are just one of several ticks that can bite humans. A common fear following a tick bite is wondering whether you are going to get Lyme disease. Because only a blacklegged tick bite can result in Lyme disease, one way to tell whether you are at risk is to identify the tick. The first thing you should do is keep the tick that bit you and put it in a plastic bag containing a small piece of a tissue paper with a drop of water. The water will prevent the tick from drying out, which makes testing more difficult. Some labs will offer to test the tick to see if it is infected with *B. burgdorferi*. You can also show it to someone familiar with ticks and have it identified that way. But the best way to identify the tick is to do it yourself! In order to do so, you will need to know what other ticks exist and learn the major differences between them.

The American dog tick, known as *Dermacentor variabilis* in the science community, is a very well-known tick in all areas where Lyme disease can be found. A similar tick, called the Rocky Mountain wood tick, or *Dermacentor andersoni*, is found on the West Coast. These ticks prefer areas with little tree cover and are often found in tall grass and along walkways and trails. Larvae and nymphs of these ticks rarely bite people; usually adults are the main culprits and they are active from April to early August. Both males and females are brownish in appearance but have very distinct white patterns on the abdomen, making them rather easy to recognize. They are also larger than blacklegged ticks. Although their bites cannot cause Lyme disease, they can lead to other diseases such as Rocky Mountain spotted fever. Rocky Mountain spotted fever is a very serious disease and in some instances, can even be fatal.

 Fact

Rocky Mountain spotted fever got its name from where it was first characterized at the beginning of the last century. Rocky Mountain spotted fever does not occur only in the Rocky Mountains, however, but is much more widespread. In reality, it occurs throughout the region where American dog ticks and Rocky Mountain wood ticks are found.

The lone star tick, or *Amblyomma americanum*, has become especially abundant on the East Coast in the past few decades. Whereas fifty years ago this tick was found mainly in the South, it can now be found all the way up to Maine. Although lone star ticks cannot transmit *B. burgdorferi*, they can transmit other diseases such as ehrlichiosis and the recently discovered Heartland virus.

The lone star tick larvae come out from July to September, the nymphs from May to August, and the adults from April to August. All stages can bite people. Lone star ticks are found in the very same wooded areas as blacklegged ticks, and both species can be found on the same portion of vegetation.

In comparison to the blacklegged ticks, lone star ticks are faster and more aggressive. You can occasionally see adults of this tick rapidly crawling toward you, something that is rarely seen with blacklegged ticks. Adult lone star ticks look quite different from blacklegged ticks, so if you look closely, it should not be too difficult to distinguish between the two. The female lone stars are larger than blacklegged female adults, and they are brown in appearance with a very characteristic white dot in the middle of their abdomen. The brownish males are smaller than the females, but still bigger than the dark blacklegged males.

🅴❗ Alert

The bites of lone star ticks have also been associated with the development of a meat allergy.

The adult lone star, dog, and blacklegged ticks are relatively easy to tell apart by their size and color. However, most cases of Lyme disease are caused by the bites of blacklegged tick nymphs. The nymphs and adults of lone star and American dog ticks are out at the same time as the blacklegged tick nymphs, and are unfortunately more difficult to tell apart. Although it is possible if you really study them (blacklegged nymphs are smaller and darker than the more oval lone star and dog tick nymphs), most people have trouble distinguishing them. If you get bitten by a nymphal tick and want to know if it is a blacklegged tick, take a look at some photos from the Internet. If you still cannot tell if it is a blacklegged tick, bring it (in a plastic bag) to a tick researcher for examination.

🅴✴ Essential

The total geographical area where blacklegged ticks are found is called their "range."

There are other ticks with ranges that overlap with blacklegged ticks, such as the brown dog tick or the Gulf Coast tick. Brown dog ticks are found throughout the United States but are more common in the South. They are found in dog kennels as well as in and around human homes, and can spend their entire life cycle indoors. They typically bite dogs, but can occasionally bite people as well. As the name implies, the adults are brown in color. The Gulf Coast tick is found predominantly in the southeastern part of the country. The adults are brown with white patterns and can be mistaken for American dog ticks. Both ticks are rare in areas where Lyme disease is most common and transmit pathogens less frequently than lone star ticks and American dog ticks.

Where Are Ticks and Lyme Disease Found?

The blacklegged and western blacklegged ticks, like most hard ticks, typically live in the woods. They prefer a humid environment away from direct sunlight and are most likely to be found within leaf litter or at the tips of shrubs and grass, especially along trails or around the edges of the woods. As you would imagine, people with homes surrounded by woods are more likely to come in contact with ticks. Forestry workers, hunters, soldiers, farmers, hikers, and campers all have a higher risk of acquiring Lyme disease as well—basically anyone who spends a greater amount of time in the woods than the average person. People who live in a big city, on the other hand, have a low chance of coming across a tick. For example, the risk of getting Lyme disease in a place such as Manhattan is practically zero. However, that does not mean it's impossible. Even in New York City, there are wooded parks that harbor ticks.

Just because ticks are normally found in the woods doesn't mean they can't show up in your front lawn or house. Ticks can travel, sometimes over long distances, by hitching a ride on other animals such as your pets. Occasionally, a tick will grab onto an animal but drop off sometime later without feeding. For example, if your dog or cat goes out into the woods, it can pick up ticks that can then wind up on your property, or worse, in your home.

Cases of Lyme disease can be found throughout the range of the blacklegged ticks. If you look at a map of where blacklegged and western blacklegged ticks are found in the United States, it closely resembles the distribution of Lyme disease. If blacklegged or western blacklegged ticks are not present, the risk of getting Lyme disease is zero, even if you are bitten by other kinds of ticks, though you may have to worry about getting some other tick-borne disease.

In the United States, the blacklegged tick can be found throughout the eastern part of the country. There are two areas in particular where the ticks are very abundant and, just as important, they are frequently infected with *B. burgdorferi*. The first area is the Northeast, particularly as you get closer to the Atlantic Coast. The second area is the north-central part of the country, around Minnesota and Wisconsin. The northeastern and north-central areas are where the vast majority of Lyme disease cases are reported. The western blacklegged tick is found mainly along the Pacific Coast. In 2015, forty-four states reported at least one case of Lyme disease. This doesn't necessarily mean that the disease is present in all of these states; it's possible for an individual to be bitten somewhere else—while vacationing, for example— and then develop the disease after traveling home. Despite this broad distribution of cases throughout the United States, approximately 95 percent of all reported Lyme disease cases are confined to just fourteen states:

- Connecticut
- Delaware
- Maine
- Maryland
- Massachusetts
- Minnesota
- New Hampshire
- New Jersey

- New York
- Pennsylvania
- Rhode Island
- Vermont
- Virginia
- Wisconsin

The five states that typically report the highest number of cases are all in the Northeast: Connecticut, Massachusetts, New Jersey, New York, and Pennsylvania. Each of these five states typically reports between one and five thousand cases each year. However, given that the actual number of Lyme disease cases is likely about ten times higher than what is reported, these numbers are likely just a fraction of the overall cases in these states.

Blacklegged ticks and Lyme disease aren't exclusive to the United States but can also be found in Canada. Although Lyme disease is reported in Canada at a much lower frequency than in the United States, it appears that the range of blacklegged ticks is increasing in Canada, along with an increase in reports of the disease. In the early 1990s, only a small area located on the Ontario shore of Lake Erie was known to contain blacklegged ticks. Since then, however, these ticks have been found in many more provinces, such as southern Manitoba, southern and eastern Ontario, and areas in New Brunswick, Nova Scotia, and Quebec. In addition, western blacklegged ticks are found in the southern part of British Columbia. The number of reported Lyme disease cases in Canada is low compared to the number of cases in the United States (there were only 315 reported in 2012), but, as is the case in the United States, this number is very likely an underestimate.

Lyme disease is not just a North American disease. It is also found throughout Europe, across northern Asia, and in Japan. In Europe, Lyme disease is the most common disease transmitted by ticks, just like it is the United States. It is most frequent in central

Europe, with the Czech Republic, Estonia, Lithuania, and Slovenia reporting the highest number of cases. Unlike the United States, the blacklegged tick is not found in Europe. Instead, the tick responsible is the castor-bean tick, also known as *Ixodes ricinus*, while in Asia, it is the taiga tick, or *Ixodes persulcatus*.

 Alert

As in the United States, reported cases of Lyme disease in Europe have risen substantially, from around 3,000 in 1990 to about 35,000 in 2010. However, underreporting is likely also very high—so the true numbers are likely much higher!

For the past two decades, there have been claims that Lyme disease may be present in Australia as well. These claims were supported by reports published in scientific literature of over 500 cases of a Lyme-like disease being found there. However, closer examinations revealed that these diagnoses were highly questionable due to flaws in the testing processes. In addition, none of the ticks known to transmit the *Borrelia* that cause Lyme disease are found in Australia, and testing of other tick species has not identified the presence of *Borrelia* spirochetes. Based on these findings, Lyme disease is not currently recognized as being present in Australia.

The Blacklegged Tick in the Southern United States

Although blacklegged ticks are present in the southeastern and south-central United States, their life cycle and feeding habits are quite different from the ticks up north. Whereas the northern blacklegged ticks have a two-year life cycle, southern ticks can complete the entire life cycle in one year due to the difference in climate. The larval and nymphal ticks in the Northeast mainly feed on rodents, whereas the immature ticks in the Southeast prefer to feed on lizards. The lizards do not get infected by *B. burgdorferi*, which means very few southern ticks become infected with *B. burgdorferi*. In addition, for some unknown reason, southern black-legged tick nymphs rarely bite humans. Because of all these factors, Lyme disease is very rare to nonexistent in the South, even in areas where ticks may be present.

 Fact

> Because of the differences of the blacklegged ticks in the Northeast and the Southeast, at one time some researchers thought these were actually two different species of ticks, *Ixodes scapularis* in the South and *Ixodes dammini* in the Northeast. However, further research did not prove this, and since 1993, these ticks are all considered *I. scapularis*. Keep this in mind if you come across an older text that refers to *I. dammini*.

How Is Lyme Disease Transmitted?

Lyme disease is a vector-borne disease. A vector is a living organism that can transmit infectious diseases between animals and humans. Vector-borne diseases account for approximately 17 percent of all infectious diseases worldwide. Vectors such as mosquitoes, ticks, flies, sand flies, lice, and fleas are particularly important because they can all acquire a pathogen from an infected host during a blood meal and then infect new hosts during subsequent feedings. Mosquitoes are the most frequent cause of vector-borne disease worldwide. This is mostly due to the high frequency of mosquito-borne malaria, which occurs in more than 200 million people each year. However, when considering which vector can transmit the greatest overall variety of diseases, it is ticks that carry that unfortunate mantle. In the United States, where malaria is rare, Lyme disease is by far the most common vector-borne disease.

The Feeding Process

To find hosts, ticks crawl upward to the tips of grass or brush or settle on the edge of leaves on the ground. They then lift their front legs in the air and wait for any object to brush by. This tick behavior is called "questing." If a person, an animal, or even an inanimate object comes in contact with the tick, it immediately grabs on. There is a misconception that ticks, like fleas, can jump; they cannot, nor can they fly. Once a tick finds a suitable host, it crawls around for an ideal feeding spot, which can take minutes or sometimes even hours. This ideal spot may be any part of the body, although ticks generally prefer locations around the head— the ears in particular.

 Fact

When unfed, the tick body is flat. During feeding they engorge, or expand their bodies. As ticks swell up with blood (become engorged), some can increase in size up to 600-fold!

Ticks that feed in areas of the body that are difficult to check are the most worrisome. They can feed on your back, armpits, or scalp and can even crawl under a sock and feed on the soles of your feet. Once they find the right spot, they begin the feeding process. They puncture the skin by inserting a tube called a hypostome, which acts as their mouth when they feed. The hypostome has serrated edges on each side, giving it a saw-like appearance. Because of these jagged edges and a cement-like substance the tick secretes to keep it in place, the hypostome is notoriously difficult to pull out when it is embedded in the skin. Anyone who has ever tried to pull out an attached tick knows that it is a challenging task.

If I Get Bitten by a Tick, Will I Always Get Lyme Disease?

Luckily, even a bite with an infected tick doesn't necessarily result in Lyme disease. It takes anywhere from thirty-six to forty-eight hours for the bacteria to travel from the gut of the tick to the salivary glands where it can be transmitted. If, during that time, you spot the tick embedded in your skin and remove it promptly, it will not be enough time for the bacteria to get to the tick's salivary glands and you won't get infected.

Even if a blacklegged tick has fed for over forty-eight hours, the bite doesn't necessarily mean you have Lyme disease. Not all blacklegged ticks are infected with *B. burgdorferi*. Scientists who study ticks and Lyme disease estimate that approximately 5 to 25 percent of nymphs and 40 to 75 percent of adults are infected with *B. burgdorferi*, although these numbers can vary widely among different geographical regions. This means you are more likely to get Lyme disease if you are bitten by an adult rather than a nymph, simply because adults are more frequently infected. It also means that because, at most, a quarter of nymphs are infected, most bites from nymphs will not result in Lyme disease.

✅ Fact

Scientists study ticks by collecting them in a method called tick "dragging" or "flagging." They drag a strip of white corduroy cloth over vegetation that may contain ticks, allow the ticks to grab on, and then pick them off the cloth. If you see anyone dragging a white cloth over vegetation in your area, they are most likely collecting ticks.

Cycle of Infection

B. burgdorferi exist in a continuous cycle between ticks and animals. In late summer, larval blacklegged ticks are infected with

B. burgdorferi by feeding on an infected animal, usually a mouse. The following spring and early summer, as nymphs, these ticks will feed and infect another mouse. That mouse will then pass the infection to a new set of larvae that will feed on it in late summer. The cycle then continues on and on. Although blacklegged ticks can feed on a wide variety of animals, the white-tailed deer and the white-footed mouse are the most important for keeping this cycle going. Their roles are quite different, however. The white-tailed deer are necessary for maintaining a large population of blacklegged ticks in the environment, whereas the white-footed mouse is essential for continuous infection of these ticks with *B. burgdorferi*.

 Alert

Humans have no role in the life cycle of *B. burgdorferi*. Because the possibility of a person transmitting the bacteria to another host is virtually zero, we are known as "dead-end hosts." This means we cannot pass the infectious agent, in this case the bacteria *B. burgdorferi*, to another person or animal.

The White-Footed Mouse

Although there are a lot of different animals ticks can feed on in the woods, one particular mouse, called the white-footed mouse, is present throughout nearly the entire range of the blacklegged tick. The white-footed mouse is the most common rodent in the woods of the eastern United States. Because white-footed mice are the most abundant animal, they are the most frequent source of blood meals for blacklegged tick larvae and nymphs. They are also the main source of infection of blacklegged ticks with *B. burgdorferi*. Throughout the spring and summer, these mice are repeatedly bitten by blacklegged tick nymphs, to the extent that, by summer's end, most have been infected with *B. burgdorferi*. Although the infections themselves don't appear to cause disease in the mice, they can persist in them for many months. When these mice later serve as a source of blood to larvae in late summer and early fall, they pass on the infection to the larvae.

 Fact

The seasonality of the nymphs and larvae is crucial for the persistence of *B. burgdorferi* in tick populations. Because infected nymphs feed first, they will infect the mice, which in turn will infect the larvae later on. This ensures that a continuous cycle of infection occurs each year.

Scientists refer to the white-footed mouse as a "reservoir" of *B. burgdorferi*. A reservoir is any animal that acts as a continuous source of infection. There are several different animals that serve as reservoirs of *B. burgdorferi*, including chipmunks, shrews, raccoons, and other small animals. However, none of them are as efficient in infecting ticks with *B. burgdorferi* as the white-footed mouse. A blacklegged tick larva is much more likely to get infected with *B. burgdorferi* by feeding on an infected white-footed mouse than by feeding on any other infected animal. As a result, the white-footed mouse is the main reservoir of *B. burgdorferi* and the primary reason why so many ticks are infected.

Fact

Although white-footed mice do not show any disease when infected with *B. burgdorferi*, other types of mice, particularly lab mice, do. When infected with *B. burgdorferi*, these mice can even get arthritis, which scientists can diagnose by measuring the swelling in the back limbs of the mice.

Some scientists have uncovered a fascinating way acorns may indirectly affect the frequency of Lyme disease. Acorns are nuts that are produced by oak trees and serve as food for mice and other small rodents. In years where more acorns are produced, rodents such as the white-footed mouse have more food, which means more mice survive and reproduce. This means that the next year after a good acorn crop, there are substantially more mice and other small rodents around for the blacklegged ticks to feed on. This is ideal for ticks because now there are more of these animals that can serve as hosts for blood meals. More mice result in more larval ticks feeding and then, consequently, more nymphs the following year in the spring. Therefore, two years after a plentiful acorn crop, you should be wary—more ticks are going to be around!

The White-Tailed Deer

The white-tailed deer is the most common type of deer living in the eastern United States. Multiple studies have shown that there is a close connection between the presence of deer and Lyme disease. Although the deer can serve as a source of a blood meal for all three life stages of the blacklegged ticks, they are resistant to *B. burgdorferi*, meaning they do not get the disease themselves. Therefore, they cannot transmit the Lyme disease bacteria to larvae or nymphs of the blacklegged tick. The primary role of deer in the continuous cycle of Lyme disease is as a source of blood for adult female blacklegged ticks.

Adult blacklegged ticks prefer to feed on large animals and will not feed on smaller animals such as rodents or birds. Adult ticks would rather feed on animals such as deer, dogs, cats, opossums, raccoons, foxes, coyotes, or skunks. Deer, however, are by far the most frequent source of a blood meal for adult ticks. Anywhere between 50 and 95 percent of all female adult ticks get their meal from feeding on deer, and a single deer can have hundreds of adult blacklegged ticks attached to it. An increase in the number of deer typically results in an increase in the number of ticks present. The opposite is true as well: if deer are rare or absent, it will result in a huge reduction or total absence of blacklegged ticks. This is why deer are the most important host for maintaining the blacklegged tick population.

Interestingly, an increase in the deer population in the second half of the twentieth century has been directly linked to the emergence of Lyme disease. Before European colonization, there may have been over twenty million white-tailed deer in what is now the United States. However, in the eighteenth and nineteenth centuries, forests were cleared for farmland and deer were more aggressively hunted. As a result, the deer population drastically declined and in some areas was virtually eliminated. In the second half of the twentieth century, a shift away from farming resulted in substantial portions of agricultural land reverting back to woodlands. The reestablishment of forests, coupled with the reduction in hunting, allowed the deer population to quickly increase. It has been estimated that the deer population in Connecticut at the end of the nineteenth century may have been as low as twelve animals. By the year 2000, it had increased to approximately 76,000. By the latter part of the 1990s, it was estimated that there were between 16 and 17 million deer present in the United States, with perhaps up to 2 million in the Northeast alone.

 Fact

Lyme disease is a zoonotic disease. A zoonotic disease is any disease that is spread between animals and people. It is also a noncommunicable disease, or noncontagious. This means it cannot be spread from one person to another.

The timing of the surge in deer population coincided with the emergence of Lyme disease, leading to an interesting theory. Scientists believe that blacklegged ticks and deer may have been abundant prior to European colonization, but because of the near eradication of deer, blacklegged ticks may have been reduced to small, isolated patches. The subsequent boom in deer population has led to the reemergence of blacklegged ticks and Lyme disease.

Which Is More Important—Mice or Deer?

Although white-footed mice are important in continuing the cycle of infection, they are not absolutely essential. In many locations throughout the range of the blacklegged tick, other small animals such as chipmunks, shrews, skunks, and raccoons can serve as alternate hosts for *B. burgdorferi*. A fascinating example of the relationships between the blacklegged tick, white-footed mouse, and white-tailed deer was studied on Monhegan Island off the coast of Maine. Although deer and an abundant population of blacklegged ticks were present on the island, there were no white-footed mice. Instead, rats were the source of blood meals and *B. burgdorferi* for the larval and nymphal stages of the ticks. To examine the importance of deer in controlling tick populations, deer were totally removed from the island. As a result, the number of larvae and nymphs dropped drastically and were not found at all after only three years without deer on the island. Some adults were found but they were all likely imported to the island from the mainland by birds. This shows that deer are likely the more important host for blacklegged ticks.

Tick Removal

If you live in an area surrounded by woods or like to venture into the woods during the summer, it would be wise to take preventive measures against ticks throughout the year, but in particular between April and September. The best way to prevent tick bites is to avoid contact with ticks altogether. When outside, try to avoid places where ticks are typically found, such as woody or brushy areas, high grass, or leaf litter. When walking along trails, try to stay in the center of the path. Avoid wearing dark clothing because that makes it difficult to notice and remove any ticks that are crawling on you. Plain, light-colored clothing is best. Although maybe not very practical during hot summer months, long sleeves and pants are much better than shorts and short sleeves or tank tops because they expose less skin for ticks. If you are wearing pants, put your socks over the pants. After coming home, take off all your clothes and, if possible, put them in a dryer on high heat for at least ten minutes. This should kill any tick that may be hidden.

As soon as possible, perform a thorough check of your entire body. Use mirrors to examine all parts of your body, and if possible, ask your family members for help if needed. It is important to check *every* area; you never know where you might find an attached tick. Make sure you do a meticulous examination of the scalp—here you will definitely need outside help. Follow all of these measures with a shower or a bath. If you had any objects with you, such as camping gear or picnic blankets, examine them thoroughly. And of course, if you had any pets with you, check them out too. If you are a parent and your kids may have been exposed to ticks, perform this routine on your children when they get home as well.

If you do spot a tick embedded in your skin, do not panic; just remove it as soon as possible. The best and safest way to remove an attached tick is with a simple pair of fine tweezers. First, grasp the tick as close as possible to the surface of your skin and then pull upward with steady pressure. Eventually, the entire tick, including the mouth, should come out. Don't jerk or twist the tick around, nor should you just rip it out with full force. This may lead to the mouth breaking off and remaining in the skin. If this happens, use the tweezers to try to remove it as well, after cleaning the tweezers. If you aren't able to remove it, leave the mouth in the skin; it will eventually dry and fall out as the wound is healing itself. Because it is the gut, not the mouth, that contains *B. burgdorferi*, leaving the mouth in will not result in Lyme disease. Once you remove the entire tick, clean the bite area with a disinfectant such as rubbing alcohol, hydrogen peroxide, or iodine. If you do not have these, wash the bite with soap and water and then keep a close eye on it for the appearance of a rash within the next three to thirty days. Be aware that you may get a small rash, less than the size of a quarter, at the bite site due to a reaction with the tick saliva even if you're not infected with Lyme disease.

As far as the removed tick goes, *do not* crush it with the tweezers. The best thing to do is flush it down the toilet without using your hands—just drop it in while holding it with the tweezers. You can also throw it in the garbage; first stick it on some duct or Scotch tape, put it in a sealable bag, and then toss it out. Once the tick is stuck to the tape, it will not be able to escape and will just dry out and die. If you want to keep the tick for any reason, such as for lab testing, it is preferable that you just put it in a bag with a piece of wet paper or a wet cotton ball and make sure it is sealed tightly. You can put it on some tape first, but that can make it more difficult to test.

There are a number of "alternative methods" for tick removal that you may have heard about, such as putting Vaseline, nail polish, alcohol, a lit cigarette, or a hot match on the tick in order to force it to come out. *Do not* use any of these methods. Not only do they not work, but they may actually increase the chances of the tick transmitting *B. burgdorferi* to you. These methods may irritate the tick and cause it to regurgitate the contents of its gut (including the bacteria) into the wound. Tweezers are always the best choice for tick removal.

Repellants and Pesticides

Repellants and pesticides prevent bites from ticks or insects in two different ways. Repellents discourage ticks or insects from biting you. Pesticides will actively kill them. There are hundreds of different products available on the market that repel or kill ticks. Each contains some active ingredient that acts as a deterrent to the tick. Some of these active ingredients are natural, usually from a plant, while others are synthetic and produced in a lab. There are both positives and negatives with using all of these products. For example, many people are hesitant to use synthetic repellents because of potential side effects to their health. Natural repellents generally have fewer side effects than synthetic products. On the other hand, natural repellants may not provide the same level of protection. It is up to you to decide which one you are more comfortable with.

Prior to using any kind of repellent or pesticide, carefully read and follow all directions printed on the label. The label contains important information on how to properly apply the product. Some products can be applied to the skin, others only to clothing. There may be special instructions for application on children. The label will also list all the potential health hazards. These will allow you to determine if this is the product you want to use. To avoid side effects from improper use, parents should always be the ones who apply tick repellents to their kids.

✅ Fact

DEET is *not* DDT, the controversial pesticide that was frequently used in the twentieth century. DDT was banned in the United States in 1972.

DEET is probably the most famous repellent and it is the main ingredient in many frequently used anti-mosquito and tick products. DEET can come in many different concentrations. It is generally sold in sprays or lotions at concentrations between 5 and 100 percent. The CDC recommends using repellents with at least 20 percent DEET on exposed skin. Typically, the higher the concentration, the higher the level of protection.

Although DEET is very good as a repellent, you should avoid prolonged exposure—it is recommended that you wash it off immediately after coming indoors. Despite its frequent usage, the instances of side effects are relatively few. Occasionally, products that contain DEET may cause redness, rashes, or some swelling if they're left on the skin for too long. Also, they may cause pain and irritation if they get into your eyes, and if they're swallowed they may cause nausea and vomiting.

Other frequently used synthetic repellents include picaridin and IR3535. Like DEET, they are both recommended by the CDC to be used directly on your skin at a concentration of at least 20 percent. If you prefer natural compounds, oil of lemon eucalyptus is an effective repellent, although it needs to be reapplied frequently because it doesn't offer long-lasting protection.

 Fact

Permethrin isn't just used to prevent tick and insect bites. Some permethrin products are used to treat other infections caused by arthropod bites, such as scabies and head lice.

Permethrin is a pesticide that kills ticks (and insects) that come in direct contact with it. You should only use products containing permethrin on your clothes, never on your skin. Treat your clothes and any potential gear that ticks could possibly get onto with products containing 0.5 percent permethrin. Make sure to do this in a well-ventilated area, preferably outside your home, and then allow it to dry. Permethrin will continue to kill any insects or ticks even through multiple washings, and if clothing is not washed, it can remain effective for up to two weeks. You should keep any clothing treated with permethrin in a plastic bag when you're not wearing it as prolonged exposure may cause side effects. Be careful when you're using a product with permethrin. It can cause eye irritation, particularly if directions on the label have not been followed.

Keeping Ticks Away from Your Property

If you live near the woods, ticks can often be found at the edge of your property and occasionally on your property itself. There are several simple things homeowners can do to reduce the likelihood of getting bitten by ticks on their property. First, properties that are overgrown with weeds or tall grass encourage tick-harboring rodents such as the white-footed mouse. To discourage rodents, keep the lawn mowed and trim all vegetation back from the edge of your property. Remove any clutter or leaf litter, and seal any potential entry points for rodents to get into your home. If possible, put up fencing to keep out deer that can bring adult ticks onto your property. Although it might not be possible to create a 100 percent tick-free property when you live by the woods, these few simple steps will go a long way to reduce the tick population around your home.

Summary

The best way to prevent Lyme disease is to prevent tick bites. Of the approximately ninety tick species present in the United States, there are only two that can transmit *B. burgdorferi*. Over 95 percent of Lyme disease cases are caused by bites of *Ixodes scapularis*, also called the blacklegged tick or the deer tick. This tick is present nearly throughout the eastern part of the United States but is most abundant in the northeastern and north-central areas of the country, where the majority of Lyme disease infections occur. These ticks most often feed on mice and deer, which are important in maintaining a large population of infected ticks. In the West, Lyme disease is caused by bites of *Ixodes pacificus*, or the western blacklegged tick. Because of different feeding habits, very few western blacklegged ticks are infected with *B. burgdorferi*, which results in less than 5 percent of Lyme disease cases being reported in the West.

Both species of blacklegged ticks are part of a large group of ticks called hard ticks, which have three life stages: the larva, the nymph, and the adult. The nymph is the most important stage for Lyme disease transmission. The small size of the nymphs, as well as the time of the year they come out to feed, makes them ideal for transmitting *B. burgdorferi*. However, because the majority of the ticks are not infected and it takes about forty-eight hours for the bacteria to be transmitted, not all tick bites will result in Lyme disease. In order to prevent tick bites, there are a number of precautions that you can take, including using repellents and wearing clothing that minimizes tick exposure. In the event of a tick bite, prompt removal is necessary to limit the possibility of *B. burgdorferi* transmission.

CHAPTER 3

Signs and Symptoms

Lyme disease is associated with a particular set of signs and symptoms. Knowing how to recognize them can help you determine if you may, in fact, have Lyme disease. The signs and symptoms can also assist your doctor in making the correct diagnosis. The most common sign of Lyme disease is an infamous rash that appears around the tick bite. There are, however, numerous other manifestations of Lyme disease that you might not be as familiar with. In this chapter, you will learn more about the signs and symptoms associated with Lyme disease in order to know what to expect if you get bitten by an infected tick.

Stages of the Symptoms

Lyme disease has a number of signs and symptoms that can appear at different times during the course of the disease. Based on their appearance and when they occur, the progress of Lyme disease can be divided into three stages. The first stage is called the "early localized" stage, and it is characterized by the appearance of a rash at the site of the tick bite as well as some flu-like symptoms. This stage is called "localized" because the majority of *B. burgdorferi* are still concentrated within the rash site and usually have not yet infected other parts of your body. At this point, diagnosis and treatment is crucial because it may prevent further progress of the disease and the appearance of more severe symptoms later on.

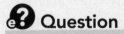 **Question**

What exactly constitutes a sign or a symptom of a disease?
Signs of a disease are characteristics that your doctor can observe or measure whereas *symptoms* are abnormalities that you feel and can tell your doctor about. For example, a runny nose is a sign of a cold while fatigue would be a symptom. Your doctor will use all of the signs and symptoms you have to make a diagnosis.

If you do not get treated during the early localized stage, the disease can progress to what is called the "early disseminated" stage. This stage is called "disseminated" because by this point, the bacteria has moved through your skin, entered your bloodstream, and spread to different parts of your body away from the site of the initial infection. The signs and symptoms associated with this stage usually appear about a month after the initial tick bite. The early disseminated stage of Lyme disease is much more serious than the early localized stage and can result in disease in different parts of your body. At this stage, *B. burgdorferi* can invade the central nervous system, heart, liver, eyes, muscles, and joints. The symptoms associated with the bacteria reaching these different organs and systems can be severe; you may suffer from intense headaches, shooting pain, facial paralysis, chest pain, and heart palpitations. Fortunately, antibiotic treatment is also effective if you are diagnosed at this stage.

The start of the last stage, called "late Lyme disease," can vary considerably among patients, but it typically occurs months after the early localized stage. Late Lyme disease is perhaps the most well-known stage of Lyme disease and is characterized by persistent attacks of arthritis. This arthritis, if not treated, can continue for weeks, months, or even years. As with the previous stages, antibiotics are the standard treatment for this stage. This treatment is usually effective; however, the time until the patient feels well again can take many months.

Although the progress of Lyme disease can be distinguished into different stages, signs and symptoms of one stage can frequently be present during the subsequent stage. For example, by the time *B. burgdorferi* have dispersed throughout the body, the initial rash may still be present along with the flu-like symptoms. Therefore, the signs and symptoms of one stage of Lyme disease do not just disappear when the next stage begins. It's more of a gradual shift, and it starts with the appearance of additional, and often more severe, signs and symptoms. In addition, some patients do not have any signs or symptoms of early localized disease, and are diagnosed only after the appearance of symptoms typical of later stages.

Erythema Migrans, or the "Bull's-Eye" Rash

The proper scientific name for the rash associated with Lyme disease is "erythema migrans" (abbreviated to EM rash from now on). This rash is the most well-known sign of Lyme disease.

The EM rash begins at the site of the tick bite; this is where the tick injected the bacteria into your skin. The appearance of the rash is usually a very unpleasant surprise given that only about a quarter of patients with Lyme disease recall being bitten by a tick before the rash appears. This is because of the location on the body where the bites that result in infection typically occur. Although the EM rash can appear anywhere on the body, there are certain parts where it is most frequently found. If a tick attaches in an area where it is easily noticeable, you will usually quickly remove it. On the other hand, attaching in a spot where it may not be seen could allow the tick to feed long enough to infect you with *B. burgdorferi*. Areas on the thigh, back, shoulder, calf, buttocks, and groin are frequent locations where EM rashes occur. Occasionally, the engorged tick can still be found in the same spot where the rash appears.

Not all EM rashes look the same but you'll often hear people describing the EM rash as having a clearing around the center, giving it a target-like or bull's-eye appearance. Because of this, the EM rash is frequently referred to as a "bull's-eye" rash. Although EM rashes indeed often have this bull's-eye appearance, most do not. For example, some do not have a central clearing, and the entire rash appears red. Therefore, you need to be aware that a rash that does not have a bull's-eye appearance can also be an EM rash.

ⓔ❋ Essential

There is a big misconception over how often the EM rash tends to appear as a "bull's-eye." Contrary to popular belief, it may only appear as a "bull's-eye" less than half the time. For this reason, calling it a "bull's-eye" rash is not really appropriate.

Although it might be the most famous sign, the EM rash doesn't necessarily appear on everyone who gets Lyme disease. It only appears on roughly three quarters of people infected with *B. burgdorferi*. It doesn't occur immediately after the tick bite. Generally, it takes between three days and a month after the initial bite for the rash to appear. Most patients get it after about one week. In cases where multiple tick bites occurred, you might find more than one rash, sometimes even crossing over each other.

The EM rash typically begins with a small raised bump or swelling at the site of the tick bite. As it begins to expand, the central tick-bite area may stay slightly raised. Over the following days, the rash expands outward, giving it a round shape. Most EM rashes are usually between four and six inches in diameter, but can be as large as twenty-eight inches.

As the rash expands, it is usually not itchy or painful, but may feel warm to the touch. It usually lasts for around three to five weeks, but not always; it can last for as little as a day. Although the round shape is most common, the shape of the rash is often based on the area of the body where it occurs. Occasionally it may appear in an unusual shape, such as a triangle, as the bacteria move over skin folds in the groin area, for instance. However, even if you miss the rash and go without treatment, the initial rash will usually resolve itself within about four weeks.

 Alert

> The rash is a result of inflammation—it is our immune system reacting to the *B. burgdorferi* moving through the skin away from the site of the tick bite.

The EM rash doesn't appear in all patients with Lyme disease. If you experience other symptoms you're going to read about later in this chapter, the absence of a rash does not mean you don't have the disease. In addition, some individuals may have had an EM rash but were not aware of it, particularly if it appeared in an area of the body where the rash was not easily noticed, such as on the scalp.

Secondary Rashes

If not treated quickly, many people with Lyme disease can develop secondary rashes. These secondary rashes, also called EM rashes, are similar to the initial rash but are usually smaller. Unlike the initial EM rash, they are not caused by a tick bite and lack the small bump at the center. These secondary rashes are caused by the bacteria invading new sites in the skin. Once *B. burgdorferi* has successfully migrated away from the site of the initial tick bite, it will eventually enter the bloodstream, where it can then be carried to different parts of the body, leave the bloodstream, and once again move through the skin. Each secondary rash represents a different group of *B. burgdorferi* that has been transported through the bloodstream and begun moving through the skin again.

The development of secondary rashes is not uncommon and can occur in up to half of all untreated cases of Lyme disease. The number of secondary rashes that appear varies from patient to patient, but generally ranges between one or two secondary rashes to well over twenty or thirty. Still, like the initial rash, these secondary rashes will eventually disappear after a few weeks.

Similar Non-EM Rashes

Various rashes that appear on your body that are not caused by an infection with *B. burgdorferi* may be mistaken for an EM rash. Rashes due to a ringworm infection (a fungal infection) are circular in appearance and also have a central clearing. However, ringworm rashes develop much more slowly than an EM rash, typically in weeks rather than days. Unlike an EM rash, ringworm rashes also appear scaly and irregular, with the borders of the rash raised relative to the skin. Many insect and tick bites can also result in the development of a rash, mainly due to a reaction with the arthropod's saliva. These rashes appear quickly, sometimes while a tick is still attached. Because it takes about two days for *B. burgdorferi* to be transmitted, a quick rash appearing at the bite site is usually not an EM rash. One way to differentiate these rashes from an actual EM rash is to compare the size. For the rash to be a sign of Lyme disease, it has to have a diameter of at least two inches. Rashes caused by insect bites are usually less than two inches and disappear quickly, within twenty-four to forty-eight hours.

Skin conditions such as cellulitis or shingles may also resemble an EM rash. However, rashes associated with cellulitis tend to look more band-like, whereas shingles rashes have large bumps throughout the rash. Because there are so many rashes that may look like an EM rash, if you happen to get a rash that you think may be an EM rash, talk to your doctor before assuming you have Lyme disease.

⊛ Essential

There is a tick-bite–related illness called southern tick-associated rash illness, or STARI, that is characterized by a rash similar to an EM rash. The two rashes are so similar that even doctors have trouble distinguishing the two, and both are likely to be treated with antibiotics. However, STARI is not Lyme disease and is not caused by blacklegged tick bites. For more information about STARI, take a look at Appendix C: Infections Transmitted by Other Ticks.

Other Symptoms of Early Localized Lyme Disease

Along with the appearance of an EM rash, Lyme disease often begins with the appearance of a wide range of symptoms that are similar to the flu, such as a fever, chills, headache, sweats, muscle aches, joint pain, fatigue, and swollen lymph nodes. Less frequently, you may experience nausea, dizziness, loss of concentration, and red eyes. Although these symptoms are considered "flu-like," symptoms such as a runny nose, sore throat, or cough are not associated with Lyme disease, which is one way the symptoms of Lyme disease can be differentiated from an actual flu.

These symptoms usually occur at the same time as the EM rash. In some cases, they may start before the appearance of the rash or after it disappears. Some people may think that the absence of the EM rash indicates that these flu-like symptoms are the result of some other infection, and may not seek treatment. Therefore, be aware that the EM rash and the flu-like symptoms are not dependent on each other.

Lyme Neuroborreliosis

When *B. burgdorferi* spreads from the site of the tick bite and infects the central nervous system, it can cause a variety of neurological signs and symptoms that are all collectively called Lyme neuroborreliosis. Lyme neuroborreliosis is the most common symptom of the early disseminated stage of Lyme disease. Neuroborreliosis itself can be divided into early and late stages, depending on how long a person has had neurological symptoms.

ⓔ❓ Question

What does "neuroborreliosis" mean?

"Neuro" is a prefix relating to your central nervous system and "borreliosis" simply means an infection from the *Borrelia* bacteria. Therefore, neuroborreliosis refers to an infection of the nervous system by *Borrelia*. The term "Lyme" is added to specify that it is caused by *Borrelia burgdorferi* specifically.

Early Neuroborreliosis

Early Lyme neuroborreliosis usually begins about one month after the initial appearance of the EM rash. On rare occasions, it can develop much earlier, perhaps within a week of the initial infection. The rash may still be present when the neurologic symptoms begin. The majority of neuroborreliosis cases occur in the summer and early fall and are most often diagnosed in children, followed by adults over fifty years old. It doesn't occur in all untreated patients—only about 15 percent of patients with untreated Lyme disease develop this condition. However, a quick diagnosis and antibiotic treatment during the early localized stage reduce the chance of developing neuroborreliosis to less than 2 percent.

Three different neurological conditions are usually found in neuroborreliosis patients: facial palsy, meningitis, and radiculoneuritis.

Because they are the conditions most frequently seen, they are often called the triad of neuroborreliosis. All three of these conditions may occur alone or at the same time as one another.

Facial Palsy

In the United States, the development of facial palsy is the most frequent sign of neuroborreliosis. Facial palsy occurs when the main nerves that are responsible for controlling facial movements are "choked," probably due to swelling around them. As a result, if you develop this condition, you may be unable to move the portion of your face that is affected, which typically will be an entire half of your face. If you look in the mirror, half of your face will appear normal while the other half will look paralyzed and appear droopy. You may have difficulty forming normal facial expressions such as smiling, have difficulty with speech, and be unable to blink on the affected side.

 Essential

Some people think that the appearance of facial palsy is a sign of a stroke. A stroke is a severe condition that results from not enough blood reaching the brain, and can also appear as a numbness or weakness in one side of the body. However, a stroke that affects facial muscles would likely affect other parts of the body as well, as opposed to a facial palsy that only affects the face.

The majority of diagnosed cases of facial palsy in the United States are not related to Lyme disease, and are usually called Bell's palsy. Neuroborreliosis patients with facial palsy can frequently be misdiagnosed as having non-Lyme–related Bell's palsy, especially if they don't have other symptoms, as is sometimes the case. However, in areas where Lyme disease is common, neuroborreliosis may be the cause of up to 25 percent of all adult facial palsy. In addition, a condition called bilateral facial palsy, when both sides of the face may be affected within days of each other, is common with Lyme neuroborreliosis, but not with Bell's palsy. Fortunately, facial palsy due to neuroborreliosis is not permanent and typically will resolve itself over time, even without treatment.

 Fact

Scientists believe that the main cause of Bell's palsy in people is herpes simplex virus 1, the primary cause of cold sores.

Meningitis

The meninges are three layers of tissue surrounding the brain and spinal column, which are the main components of the central nervous system. The main function of the meninges is to protect the central nervous system. Cerebrospinal fluid, a clear, colorless fluid that acts as a cushion for the brain, is found within the meninges.

 Fact

Many different microorganisms besides *B. burgdorferi* can cause meningitis. Probably the most common cause of meningitis are certain types of viral infections that cause mild symptoms that resolve within a few days. Other agents, particularly bacteria, can cause severe, life-threatening meningitis.

In the early disseminated phase of Lyme disease, *B. burgdorferi* may infect the meninges, resulting in swelling. This condition is called meningitis. Meningitis caused by Lyme disease is characterized by headaches that range in intensity from mild to absolutely disabling. The pain is typically specific to a particular section of the head, usually either the front or the back, but it can also be more generalized. About one quarter of patients with Lyme meningitis also have mild neck stiffness. Some patients experience nausea, vomiting, and light sensitivity, although these symptoms are less frequent. The symptoms of Lyme meningitis can continue for weeks or months if not treated.

ⓔ Alert

Meningitis is not the infection of the brain itself, which is called encephalitis. Because each affects the central nervous system, they are both serious conditions. Encephalitis can sometimes occur in Lyme disease patients with late neuroborreliosis, especially in Europe.

Radiculoneuritis

Radiculoneuritis occurs when *B. burgdorferi* affects the nerve roots at the spot where they connect to the spine. The resulting inflammation can cause sharp stabbing, burning, or shooting pains that travel down into the arms or torso. Occasionally, patients may have difficulty with movement. The pain can be severe, deep in the muscle, and usually increases at night. Some people also experience numbness or tingling in their hands.

Late Neuroborreliosis

Late neuroborreliosis occurs much less frequently than early neuroborreliosis. In late neuroborreliosis, the neurological disease has been going on for more than six months. Very few individuals with late neuroborreliosis have been examined by doctors, mainly because most patients are treated before the development of this condition.

In addition to experiencing symptoms of the early stages of the disease, such as body aches or fatigue, patients with late neuroborreliosis usually suffer from a variety of cognitive problems involving their memory, learning, perception, and problem solving. The most commonly reported cognitive problem in these patients is short-term memory loss. They also may have difficulty with finding the right word and concentrating. Normal everyday tasks may become more difficult and take longer to complete, and some patients may experience psychiatric problems. They may have drastic mood changes and be irritable, emotional, highly anxious, or depressed. They may become extra sensitive to sound. Patients who have late Lyme neuroborreliosis have also reported sleep disturbances, including the need for extra hours of sleep.

Lyme Carditis

Another condition associated with the early disseminated stage is called Lyme carditis, which occurs when *B. burgdorferi* invades the heart. It is estimated that approximately 5 to 10 percent of untreated individuals with Lyme disease develop this condition. It was reported more frequently in the mid-1980s; nowadays, with improvements in earlier diagnosis and treatment, Lyme carditis is rare. Between 2001 and 2010, just slightly over 1 percent of Lyme disease cases included any symptoms associated with the heart. Both adults and children can develop Lyme carditis, but cases have been more frequently diagnosed in adults and more often in men.

The symptoms of Lyme carditis usually begin about two to five weeks after the appearance of an EM rash, although they may occur as quickly as two days or as many as seven months after the infection begins. You may still have signs and symptoms from the early localized stage, such as a fever or a rash, when Lyme carditis begins to appear, and it is possible to have Lyme carditis at the same time as Lyme neuroborreliosis.

The most common manifestation of Lyme carditis is a disorder called "heart block." Heart block is an abnormal condition where the heart beats too slowly. A normal heartbeat is coordinated by electrical signals sent from the upper part (called the atrium) of the heart to the lower part (called the ventricles). When *B. burgdorferi* enters the heart, it causes inflammation that can partially or totally block the movement of these electrical signals. This blockage prevents a normal heartbeat. Symptoms of heart block can include light-headedness, palpitations, shortness of breath, chest pain, and fainting.

Heart block can fluctuate in severity between mild, moderate, and severe, and can quickly progress through the stages. In a mild heart block, the electrical signals are slowed but reach the lower part of the heart. Mild heart block rarely causes problems and generally no treatment is required. In moderate heart block, the signals are slowed even more, and some can't reach the ventricles. In severe heart block, none of the signals reach the ventricles and heart failure could result. In cases of moderate and severe heart block, you need to go to the hospital immediately, especially because the severity of the block can quickly change. Cases of moderate and especially severe heart block might require a doctor to put in a temporary pacemaker to make sure your heart beats properly. Because Lyme carditis can be treated, you shouldn't need a permanent pacemaker.

Although Lyme disease can be a severe illness, it is rarely fatal. However, there have been several reports of death due to Lyme carditis. According to the CDC, between 1985 and 2014, there have been ten deaths out of approximately seventeen hundred cases of Lyme carditis reported in the United States. The fatal cases all occurred in areas where Lyme disease is common and occurred in adults of all ages, including some in their twenties and thirties. The patients collapsed suddenly due to heart failure and were unable to be resuscitated. Many of these patients had an illness in the weeks before they collapsed, which likely was undiagnosed Lyme disease. Others had known exposure to ticks. None of these fatal Lyme carditis patients were probably even aware that they had Lyme disease.

Lyme Arthritis

The onset of arthritis is the hallmark of late Lyme disease. Months to years after the initial infection, more than half of untreated patients develop recurring episodes of joint pain and swelling. When Lyme disease was first discovered, arthritis was the primary symptom associated with this illness. This is not the case today, and Lyme arthritis is much rarer now than it was in the past. People who live in Lyme disease–endemic areas are much more aware of Lyme disease than they were thirty to forty years ago, and most get treated before the disease progresses to the arthritis stage. Today, the majority of patients who develop Lyme arthritis only progress that far because they did not have any prior symptoms and were not even aware they had the disease in the first place.

🅔✷ Essential

The swelling and pain in the joints in the late arthritis stage of Lyme disease is caused by a massive inflammatory response of our immune system to the presence of *B. burgdorferi*.

Early in the course of Lyme disease, *B. burgdorferi* can migrate to joints, tendons, or bursas, which are fluid-filled sacs in joints that reduce friction. At this point, most patients typically do not have any symptoms of arthritis, although some may have joint pain. If the disease is left untreated, months later it will eventually progress to the late Lyme arthritis stage. All other signs and symptoms of Lyme disease are typically gone by this stage of the illness. If you develop Lyme arthritis, you may experience brief, recurring attacks of swelling and pain in either a single or multiple joints. Arthritis is most often found in the knees, which can become very swollen and may feel warm to the touch. Other joints that are frequently affected include shoulders, ankles, elbows, or wrists. Even if you have pain in multiple joints, it will usually be fewer than five. The swelling may affect your range of motion, and many patients can-not put any weight on the affected joint. Some patients may have permanent joint destruction. The progress of Lyme arthritis is slow, and it may be years into the infection before irreversible damage occurs in the joints. Lyme arthritis can be successfully treated with antibiotics, which we'll discuss in Chapter 6.

Over time, both the frequency and severity of arthritis attacks decline. Even in patients not treated with antibiotics, arthritis, like other signs and symptoms of Lyme disease, will eventually go away. However, for some people, arthritis continues for years and does not go away, even after long-term antibiotic treatments. This condition is called "antibiotic-refractory Lyme arthritis." Although the cause of this condition is unknown, there are several possible explanations. One possibility is that the development of this condition may depend on the type of *B. burgdorferi* strain you are infected with. Some strains of *B. burgdorferi* tend to cause a higher degree of inflammation in the host than others. Another possibility is that perhaps patients with this condition cannot clear dead bacteria from their body for some unknown reason. However, the immune system continuously tries to attack the dead bacteria, and this results in persistent inflammation. Other possible explanations may include genetic factors specific to the person, such as the development of an autoimmune disease, which results in constant inflammation. Some or all of these factors may contribute to the development of antibiotic-refractory Lyme arthritis. However, even in individuals with this condition, the symptoms of arthritis eventually do resolve with time, although it may take years.

Not all untreated patients with Lyme disease will develop Lyme arthritis. The reasons for this are not known, but again, it is likely that genetic differences, both in *B. burgdorferi* and the host, may play a role. Given that there is a large difference in the ability of various *B. burgdorferi* strains to cause severe disease throughout the body, it seems probable that infection with less pathogenic strains of *B. burgdorferi* may be less likely to cause arthritis. In addition, genetic factors in different individuals may help their immune system limit the development of Lyme arthritis.

Lyme Disease in Europe

In Europe, Lyme disease is caused by three different species of *Borrelia* bacteria: *B. afzelii, B. garinii,* and *B. burgdorferi.* Although all three species may cause an EM rash, disease with each species tends to follow a different pattern after that. Just like in the United States, the European *B. burgdorferi* causes arthritis in the late stage of Lyme disease. *B. afzelii* and *B. garinii*, however, are rarely associated with arthritis. Instead, infection with *B. garinii* generally leads to a higher risk of neuroborreliosis, which is two to five times more likely to occur with *B. garinii* than with the other two species. Untreated late-stage infections with *B. afzelii* can cause a skin condition not seen with either *B. burgdorferi* or *B. garinii* called acrodermatitis chronica atrophicans (abbreviated to ACA) that leads to inflammation, swelling, and bluish-red lesions on the hands and feet. ACA is unusual in that it is the only aspect of Lyme disease that does not resolve itself over time and causes permanent death of the affected skin.

🚫 Alert

Remember, you can get Lyme disease outside of the United States. If you plan to go on a European vacation and expect to be doing any outdoor recreational activities such as camping or hiking, you need to take the same precautions against tick bites as you would in North America.

Reinfection

Lyme disease is not a one-time-only disease. Even if you already had Lyme disease, any exposure to ticks leaves you vulnerable to getting reinfected. A reinfection occurs when you get bitten by a *B. burgdorferi*-infected tick some time after the completion of successful treatment for the initial bout of the disease. A reinfection is not a relapse, but is a new infection with *B. burgdorferi* that may lead to a different set of symptoms, depending on the strain.

Reinfection is not a rare occurrence; between 1 and 15 percent of people with Lyme disease are reinfected within the next five years. In a study that followed Lyme disease patients over one to two decades, nearly a quarter of the patients reported a second infection. So why do you get reinfected? Why aren't people immune following the initial infection?

Many people with Lyme disease live in areas where they are frequently exposed to ticks. It is very likely that this continuous exposure will lead to repeated tick bites. In one study that looked at tick bites in New York State, nearly 18 percent of people reported new bites within six weeks of their initial bite. Even though you do generate some degree of immunity from your initial bout of Lyme disease, it unfortunately does not fully protect you against a reinfection. This is especially true if you get infected with a strain of *B. burgdorferi* that is different from the strain that was responsible for the initial infection. It has been shown that patients who experience reinfection are almost always infected by a different strain. To make matters worse, the immunity you acquire to the initial strain may wane over time. Typically, in about six years, it will weaken enough so that you may get reinfected with the initial strain.

Reinfection is much more likely to occur in Lyme disease patients who were successfully treated in the early stage of the disease, for example, soon after the appearance of an EM rash. Conversely, reinfection is extremely unlikely to occur in Lyme disease patients who progressed to late Lyme disease. This is because the ability of your immune system to fight off *B. burgdorferi* becomes substantially more developed as you progress further into the disease. By late Lyme disease, you will have developed a very strong immune response that is much more likely to prevent a subsequent *B. burgdorferi* infection, even if it is caused by a different strain.

Summary

The course of Lyme disease is often divided into three stages, which are called early localized, early disseminated, and late Lyme disease. The first stage of the disease most often includes the appearance of an expanding rash at the site of the tick bite, called an erythema migrans. The rash is frequently accompanied by fever, muscle aches, and other flu-like symptoms. The bacteria then spread to other parts of the body, and about a month after the initial infection, symptoms of early disseminated disease start to appear. Facial palsy, headaches, and shooting pain indicate that *B. burgdorferi* has infected the central nervous system, which is a condition called Lyme neuroborreliosis. Other times, the bacteria can infect the heart, causing Lyme carditis. Eventually, months after the initial infection, late Lyme disease begins, characterized by arthritis, especially in the knees. The disease can be treated with antibiotics at all stages, although the later in the disease the treatment begins, the longer it may take to feel better. However, in some patients with late Lyme disease, the treatment is not effective and symptoms may continue for years, even though the bacteria is not believed to be present anymore.

Patients who have had late Lyme disease appear to be resistant to another infection later on. This is in contrast to patients treated during the early localized and disseminated stages, who do not become immune to it, and if bitten by another infected tick, wind up getting the disease again.

CHAPTER 4

Complications of Lyme Disease

Among the most mysterious and troubling aspects of Lyme disease is that some symptoms of this disease can continue even after treatment with antibiotics. Ideally, you'd expect that getting a Lyme disease diagnosis and following it up with an antibiotic treatment would cause all of your disease symptoms to subside. This, unfortunately, is not the case for all people with Lyme disease. A number of patients treated for this illness continue to have persistent symptoms, in some cases for years after treatment. This condition, called posttreatment Lyme disease syndrome, has been perplexing doctors for years. What causes it? Why do some patients develop it, while others don't? And what can be done to cure it? Unfortunately, the answers to these questions are not clear. The lack of understanding of this condition, coupled with a lack of treatment options, has given rise to alternative beliefs that question what Lyme disease really is. Over the years, these beliefs have fueled a large number of controversies associated with this illness. The main dispute lies in the existence of a condition called "chronic Lyme disease" and how it actually relates to Lyme disease.

Posttreatment Lyme Disease Syndrome

In the majority of cases, if you receive a diagnosis of Lyme disease and begin treatment in the early part of the disease, your symptoms will go away within a few weeks without any long-term complications. Unfortunately, a quick diagnosis and antibiotic treatment does not guarantee an immediate return to health for everyone afflicted with Lyme disease. In some rare cases, you may continue to have symptoms even after you complete antibiotic therapy.

The types of symptoms that you may have can vary, but usually consist of fatigue, joint pain, and muscle aches. They often also include a variety of mental conditions, ranging from minor difficulties, such as an inability to concentrate, to severe problems like depression. Adding to the confusion, the timing of these symptoms can be inconsistent as well, occurring constantly in some patients while only sporadically in others. If you continue to have these symptoms after you've completed your antibiotic treatment, and they persist for at least six months, you have a condition called "posttreatment Lyme disease syndrome" (abbreviated to PTLDS). In some cases, this condition has been shown to continue for more than ten years.

Question

What is a syndrome?
A syndrome is defined as a collection of signs and symptoms that tend to occur together during a particular disease.

How Frequent Is PTLDS?

PTLDS is a confusing and complex disorder. Despite it being an area of intense research due to its mysterious nature, relatively little has been learned about this condition and its presumed link with Lyme disease. In fact, in the past there have been people who have argued that PTLDS and a prior Lyme disease infection may not even be linked. These days, it is generally accepted that PTLDS exists, although how frequently it occurs is not really clear. To use a rough estimate, approximately 10 to 20 percent of patients with Lyme disease may develop PTLDS, though some suggest that those numbers are far too low. In some communities, especially ones where Lyme disease is not diagnosed quickly, PTLDS may affect up to 50 percent of Lyme disease patients. Because many of the studies looking at PTLDS see such a wide range of symptoms, it has been very difficult to truly determine how frequently this condition occurs.

❔ Question

Do other diseases also continue to have symptoms after treatment or just Lyme disease?
No, having symptoms after completing a treatment is not unique to Lyme disease. There are other illnesses, both viral and bacterial, where it can take some time before you return to feeling normal, such as infectious mononucleosis, Q fever, and Ross River virus.

Cause of PTLDS

What causes PTLDS? The answer to that question has been eluding scientists for nearly thirty years. The short answer is nobody knows. If this syndrome was caused by *B. burgdorferi*, finding the bacteria while the person has symptoms of PTLDS would be proof of its involvement. As you will see in Chapter 5, finding *B. burgdorferi* in the patient while they have symptoms of Lyme disease is how a diagnosis of the main infection is frequently made. However, doctors and scientists haven't been able to do this with PTLDS. Because PTLDS is, by definition, *post*treatment, *B. burgdorferi* should have been eliminated and the bacteria would not be in your system. In fact, if you do have an ongoing infection with *B. burgdorferi*, you couldn't be diagnosed with PTLDS. During PTLDS, whatever damage may be occurring, an active infection with live *B. burgdorferi* is not believed to be the cause.

🅴❗ Alert

There is the possibility that *B. burgdorferi* does in fact survive after antibiotic treatment in extremely low numbers undetectable by modern science. Trying to find proof of the presence of these bacteria is extremely difficult, but is currently an area of active research.

Although it is not clear how and why PTLDS occurs, scientists do have an idea of a few potential risk factors that make it more likely for someone to develop this condition. The biggest risk factor appears to be a delay in getting diagnosed with Lyme disease, which means a later start for antibiotic treatment. PTLDS tends to occur more frequently in people who were not diagnosed in the early stages of Lyme disease. This doesn't mean that if Lyme disease is diagnosed early, you can't get PTLDS, however. Some people who do get treated early can still develop this condition. It just makes it far more likely that you'll get PTLDS if you don't get treated quickly.

There is also a link to how severe your symptoms are when you're first diagnosed. Patients with worse symptoms in the beginning stages of treatment appear to be more at risk for developing PTLDS. This is especially true for patients who developed Lyme neuroborreliosis during their initial bout with Lyme disease.

Other potential risk factors exist as well, such as a weak response of your immune system to the initial infection of Lyme disease, or improper treatment, such as using antibiotics that aren't appropriate for treating Lyme disease, which, in the long run, may actually help prolong the infection.

Although scientists still don't know exactly what causes PTLDS, they have some ideas. It's likely that the inflammation caused by your immune system to help fight off the initial infection of Lyme disease damages some parts of your body and this damage is what causes the symptoms to continue. This damage could be worse if your body develops an autoimmune response to some parts of *B. burgdorferi*. In such an event, your immune system would react as if *B. burgdorferi* were still present, even after it was cleared from your body. This has happened in other, non-Lyme disease–related infections so it seems at least plausible that it could happen here too. In addition, it appears that some people may simply be genetically predisposed to these autoimmune responses, making them more likely to develop conditions such as PTLDS. Finally, the strains of *B. burgdorferi* may also be a factor. Because certain strains can cause the symptoms of Lyme disease to be more intense and may result in more damage to your body, it's possible this damage may also lead to the symptoms of PTLDS.

ⓔ❓ Question

What exactly is an autoimmune response?
During an active infection, your immune system is turned on to fight off the bacteria. Once the bacteria are destroyed, the immune system should turn off and go back to normal. In an autoimmune response, the immune system does not fully turn off. This causes a continuous inflammation that can lead to damage inside your body and cause persistent illness.

Symptoms of PTLDS

PTLDS has a wide range of symptoms, from minor ones that won't interfere with your day-to-day life to severe problems that can greatly affect your quality of life. The main symptom, which appears in nearly every patient with PTLDS, is fatigue. Just how tired a person feels can vary and can be subjective, but about half of patients with PTLDS report feeling severe fatigue which, in some cases, may leave the patient confined to bed and unable to do anything. The fatigue is usually accompanied by muscle aches and headaches as well, with about one quarter of people who get these aches rating the pain as "severe."

More than half of PTLDS patients experience joint pain or stiffness. It's usually felt in a particular joint, such as the knee, but can occur in any joint in your body. This becomes more intense in people who progressed all the way to Lyme arthritis before they were treated. Some other symptoms that have been reported with PTLDS include shooting pains throughout the body, neck pain, a tingling sensation, and a loss of feeling in the arms, legs, hands, and face. There is also a wide range of mental problems that come along with PTLDS, such as changes in normal behavior, mood swings, and experiencing "brain fog," a difficult-to-explain condition that affects thought processes and involves an inability to focus along with a loss of memory or concentration.

Living with PTLDS

One of the most common complaints from patients with PTLDS is that the disease affects their daily life to some degree. For some patients, the symptoms are severe and affect most aspects of their everyday life. These can be both physical and psychological. Many patients with severe symptoms realize that their life is changed forever. In this new life, they have to accept that there are adjustments they will have to make in order to be able to live with their illness. Many patients are forced to give up various activities or hobbies that were part of their life prior to being diagnosed with Lyme disease. Outdoor activities, particularly ones that involve some strenuous activity such as sports or hiking, are given up. Even simpler activities that require minimal physical activity may be prohibitive. Some tasks that could be easily accomplished prior to the illness may now only be partially completed. Some patients feel that they have two lives: one before the diagnosis of Lyme disease and one after the diagnosis of Lyme disease.

PTLDS doesn't only affect a person's physical health. PTLDS can also have a substantial effect on their social and work lives. Some people are forced to give up attending various social events such as plays or ball games because they are physically unable to get through them. Problems with memory loss can affect their confidence in their social life as well as at work or school. Because PTLDS is a subjective illness, meaning there aren't any obvious and visible signs or symptoms, many patients experience a lack of understanding of their condition on the part of others. Coworkers, friends, and sometimes even family members often do not recognize the profound effect of their symptoms on their everyday life. Some patients feel they lack the support system that people with more well-known diseases such as cancer can easily obtain. Other patients find that people around them have a misunderstanding of the potential severity of Lyme disease, and they don't understand that PTLDS is a real illness where some patients don't get well right away. Some have found that their work life becomes more difficult due to supervisors not understanding their illness or disbelieving their symptoms.

People with PTLDS can also experience a tremendous amount of doubt and stress regarding their own future, not knowing whether PTLDS will be a chronic illness they have to deal with for the rest of their life. Some patients with sporadic symptoms live in constant fear that the more debilitating ones will come back or that the symptoms will get worse over time. Some individuals find themselves in fear of the woods, afraid of acquiring new tick bites and making their illness worse. There is an increase in anxiety and some patients succumb to depression, suicidal thoughts, or both.

Patients with PTLDS frequently experience frustration with doctors who have no way of understanding and treating the subjective symptoms associated with their condition. They encounter many different opinions and treatment plans offered by many different doctors, including some doctors who disbelieve the symptoms the patients claim they have. Because of the perceived lack of help from doctors, some patients undertake stronger personal responsibility for their health. For some patients, this leads to them turning to unorthodox treatments that may not be recommended by standard physicians. We discuss some of these options, both good and bad, in Chapter 6.

In addition to the human costs in suffering, PTLDS can also have a serious and negative effect on the patients' finances. Because of the severity of the symptoms, many people with PTLDS can't work full time anymore, moving to part-time work or stopping completely. Patients with PTLDS are also five times more likely to visit a doctor than regular Lyme disease patients, which, depending on their health insurance, could mean a substantial increase in out-of-pocket healthcare expenses. A recent study estimated that Lyme disease costs the US healthcare system between $712 million and $1.3 billion, or about $3,000 per patient, annually due to return doctor visits and additional testing.

How Is PTLDS Identified?

The fact that *B. burgdorferi* or any other agent hasn't yet been associated with PTLDS makes this illness very misunderstood and controversial. There are no signs of the disease that a doctor can observe. The illness is strictly subjective, with a wide range of symptoms reported by individual patients. One of the biggest struggles with PTLDS is simply identifying it in patients because there is no universally accepted definition for this condition. Even worse, there are no diagnostic tests that can clearly identify whether a patient is suffering from this illness. For most diseases, even if your signs and symptoms are not specific, diagnostic tests will usually aid your doctor in eventually reaching the correct diagnosis. There are usually some identifiers, typically found in your blood, that can be used in diagnostic tests as an indication that you have a particular illness, such as the presence of *B. burgdorferi* helping to identify Lyme disease. Although scientists are constantly looking for ways to identify PTLDS through blood samples, they haven't been able to find any yet. As a result, right now there is no test that can be used by doctors to diagnose PTLDS. So if there are no tests doctors can run and the signs and symptoms are different for each patient, how can doctors possibly diagnose this disease?

Diagnosis of PTLDS comes from the inclusion of some symptoms and factors and the exclusion of others. What does that mean exactly? Although no clear-cut definition has been given, several guidelines have been proposed that help doctors decide whether you have PTLDS. The criteria for a diagnosis of PTLDS include:

- Evidence of prior Lyme disease. This has to be documented by either a positive Lyme disease test or a diagnosis from a doctor based on the signs and symptoms, even if you were never actually tested.
- You need to have completed the antibiotic treatments and had some of the symptoms disappear as a result of that treatment. This means you did in fact get better to a certain degree after treatment.
- Within six months of the initial treatment for Lyme disease, you had to begin to feel either fatigue or muscle pain, or have some cognitive problems. These symptoms had to reduce the quality of your life in some way.

In addition to the inclusion criteria, there also exists a wide array of criteria that excludes a patient from fitting the diagnosis of PTLDS. This is meant to exclude patients who, even though they may present with similar symptoms, are more likely to be affected with some other illness. In order to be diagnosed with

PTLDS, you and your symptoms cannot fulfill any of the following criteria:

- You cannot have a diagnosis of an illness with similar symptoms. For example, if you were previously diagnosed with fibromyalgia or chronic fatigue syndrome, you will be excluded. Both of these disorders have similar symptoms to PTLDS but are not believed to be related to Lyme disease.
- You cannot have an active infection, with *B. burgdorferi* or any other pathogen. In most cases, an active infection would likely explain your symptoms instead of PTLDS.
- You cannot have symptoms that can be explained by your doctor. There may be symptoms that you believe are due to PTLDS that your doctor is able to diagnose as being caused by something else.
- You cannot have a history of unexplained symptoms before you had Lyme disease. In this case, it's likely that the current symptoms are a continuation of that earlier unknown illness.

Treatment

Unfortunately, there is no current treatment for PTLDS. Although some doctors claim that prolonged antibiotic treatment may be helpful, this is not recommended by the current treatment guidelines by the CDC. So, what to do if you have PTLDS? In most cases, a doctor can guide you on how to best manage your symptoms and reduce their effect on your everyday life. This can include prescriptions to help relieve the pain or nonpharmaceutical ways to lessen some of the symptoms such as exercise or improved nutrition.

Chronic Lyme Disease

"Posttreatment Lyme disease syndrome" is a relatively new term. Even people living in areas where Lyme disease is common have likely never heard of it. Another term, "chronic Lyme disease," is much more recognized and thought to mean the same thing as PTLDS. Chronic Lyme disease doesn't follow the same guidelines as PTLDS and so it ends up having a much more general group of people claiming they have it. Whereas PTLDS represents a group of patients who were diagnosed with Lyme disease and have clear symptoms without a sign of an active infection, chronic Lyme disease is used for individuals who claim to have some sort of a persistent active infection that is difficult to detect and cure with regular antibiotic therapy. Patients who believe they have chronic Lyme disease include a broad group of people who may suffer from a wide range of symptoms, some of which overlap with PTLDS, including chronic pain, fatigue, various cognitive problems, and behavioral changes. However, chronic Lyme disease can also overlap with a wide range of neurological and rheumatological diseases, including some that have already been described but have no known clear cause, such as multiple sclerosis or ALS, also known as Lou Gehrig's disease.

For years, the debate over the existence of chronic Lyme disease has been the focus of immense controversy and a source of disagreement fought between the scientific Lyme disease community and many individuals in the public who claim to be suffering from chronic Lyme disease. This conflict has been going on for over twenty years and has been featured on various television news programs and started countless "discussions" on the Internet. It has led to a number of multimillion-dollar lawsuits, entered the realm of politics, and even resulted in Congress holding special hearings on Lyme disease. What is the root of the disagreement? If we know that Lyme disease exists, why are people arguing about it?

The Chronic Lyme Disease Controversy

At the center of the controversy are two sides with very different opinions about what constitutes "Lyme disease." On one side are the majority of scientists and doctors, including an organization of more than nine thousand infectious disease doctors called the Infectious Diseases Society of America (IDSA). Based on all of the available clinical evidence, the IDSA has published guidelines on how to treat patients with Lyme disease. For this group, Lyme disease is defined as an infection with *B. burgdorferi* that can be cured with proper antibiotic therapy, although it is accepted that some people can develop PTLDS for an unspecified amount of time.

⚠ Alert

Lyme-literate doctors are physicians who claim to be experts in the diagnosis and treatment of patients with chronic Lyme disease. Their methods of treatment, which may include prolonged antibiotic treatment, can sometimes be at odds with the currently recommended guidelines of the larger medical community.

On the other side of the argument is a group that consists mostly of patient advocacy groups, led by the International Lyme and Associated Diseases Society (ILADS), some patients, and a small group of doctors. This side has adopted the term "chronic Lyme disease" as an explanation for a number of symptoms that involve nonspecific pain, constant fatigue, and various levels of neurocognitive problems. Members of this group often refer to themselves as "Lyme literate." They believe that Lyme disease as defined by IDSA is too limiting and does not reveal the true extent of this disease. This group has a much broader definition of Lyme disease, which includes many additional symptoms not defined by IDSA that they believe to be related to tick bites. To be diagnosed with chronic Lyme disease, a person often doesn't need to have clear evidence of a prior infection with *B. burgdorferi*. In fact, many do not. This group also believes that the antibiotic treatment guidelines recommended by the IDSA are insufficient to adequately treat this condition.

In essence, the controversy associated with chronic Lyme disease is a disagreement among these two groups as to whether chronic Lyme disease actually exists. To help you understand these differences of opinion, let's discuss different causes of the disagreements in more detail.

❓ Question

What is the International Lyme and Associated Diseases Society or ILADS?

According to their website, ILADS is a nonprofit, international, multidisciplinary medical group that seeks appropriate diagnosis and treatment of Lyme disease and Lyme disease–associated infections. The goal of ILADS is to promote the understanding of Lyme disease and associated diseases through research, education, and policy. However, in many of these areas, the perspective of ILADS is opposite the view of the Infectious Diseases Society of America.

The group championing the cause of chronic Lyme disease believes that the doses and duration of antibiotics typically prescribed for the treatment of Lyme disease are not enough to get rid of *B. burgdorferi*. They believe that a more open-ended treatment with multiple combinations of antibiotics may be necessary to totally get rid of the symptoms. The disease is also sometimes believed to be virtually incurable unless treated very early.

There are many within the chronic Lyme disease group who argue that PTLDS and chronic Lyme disease are two distinct conditions, separated by the lack of an active infection in PTLDS sufferers versus a prolonged active infection in sufferers of chronic Lyme disease. This difference is key to the argument for prolonged antibiotic treatment that has been advocated by a number of

Lyme-literate physicians. As will be discussed in Chapter 9, some studies using animals have shown that *B. burgdorferi* can sometimes remain after antibiotic treatment, which adds plausibility to this idea. In addition, *B. burgdorferi* DNA has occasionally been detected in patients long after antibiotic therapy, leading to the speculation that these people had an uncured and persistent infection such as chronic Lyme disease. One possibility put forth by the pro–chronic Lyme group is that *B. burgdorferi* can hide in certain parts of the body that antibiotics can't easily access.

Proponents of chronic Lyme disease claim that during the initial infection of Lyme disease, *B. burgdorferi* can transition from a spiral corkscrew-like shape to a different form, one that may allow the bacteria to infect human cells directly and become resistant to antibiotics. One form in particular has been detected and reported by several laboratories. This form has a round shape and has been given the various names "cyst form," "L-form," "round body," and "spheroplast." A different regimen of antibiotics is said to be needed to successfully treat this form of *B. burgdorferi*. Some also believe that *B. burgdorferi* may be able to form "biofilms," which are communities of bacteria sticking to a surface, often within a slimy-like residue that can protect them from antibiotics. These *B. burgdorferi* biofilms would then be more difficult to eradicate with standard antibiotic treatment by not allowing the antibiotics to reach all of the bacteria.

Another disagreement is with the accuracy of diagnostic testing. Chronic Lyme disease advocates claim that the diagnostic tests for Lyme disease are inadequate, and the standard blood tests recommended for Lyme disease diagnosis have little usefulness. They point to the fact that, when standard blood tests are used, some patients continuously test negative even though they previously had an EM rash diagnosed by a doctor. This has led to many alternative tests for Lyme disease being used by Lyme-literate doctors.

People with chronic Lyme disease also say that they are frequently coinfected by other pathogens. Certainly, many ticks can harbor multiple pathogens so coinfections aren't uncommon. We discuss many of them in Chapter 8. However, these coinfections don't necessarily have to be transmitted by ticks; some of them can be sexually transmitted. In addition, some believe that in addition to being transmitted by ticks, *B. burgdorferi* can also be sexually transmitted. A new term, multiple systemic infectious disease syndrome (MSIDS), has even been created to include patients that may have multiple infections with various viruses, parasites, fungi, spirochetes, and other bacteria. This promotes the idea that the symptoms of chronic Lyme disease are caused not just by a *B. burgdorferi* infection but by these coinfections, many of which are not even transmitted by ticks. It is believed by some in the chronic Lyme disease community that a combination of these infections produces toxins that cause increased inflammation and lower the ability of the immune system to fight infections.

It has also been suggested that Lyme disease may have a link to a number of other conditions not normally associated with it, including autism, Parkinson's disease, multiple sclerosis, ALS, birth defects, Alzheimer's disease, and homicidal behavior.

The Other Side of Chronic Lyme Disease

Many of these ideas are appealing because they could be used to explain the health problems of the afflicted individuals. However, the scientific community disagrees with many of these claims, primarily because many of the theories proposed by the chronic Lyme disease group lack any scientific evidence. Some of them have been actively disproved.

Scientists have performed multiple large studies to see if persistent symptoms of Lyme disease were improved by longer treatments of antibiotics, which we will go over in more detail in Chapter 6. However, the results of these studies showed that there is no significant benefit in these longer treatments. Even if some slight benefits are there, they may be outweighed by the risks of side effects of these continuous antibiotic treatments. Right now, the scientific community has found no convincing evidence that these extended treatments are helpful or that a persistent infection is responsible for the lingering symptoms after antibiotic treatment.

Another argument made by the pro–chronic Lyme disease side is that *B. burgdorferi* DNA has been found in patients after antibiotic treatment, which is true. What is unclear, however, is whether the DNA is from *live* bacteria or whether these traces consisted of dead bacteria left behind after the antibiotics and immune system killed them. If DNA from live bacteria is detected, it means that there is an active infection, which would lend credence to the claims of the pro–chronic Lyme side that *B. burgdorferi* isn't completely killed by antibiotics. Detection of DNA from dead bacteria would mean that the infection *was* eradicated by the initial antibiotic treatment. Live bacteria have been found in animals following antibiotic treatment, but these bacteria are different from the original infecting strain, and their ability to cause any disease is questionable.

There is no evidence that other forms of *B. burgdorferi*, including the round "cyst forms," occur in people. A number of sophisticated Lyme disease laboratories have never detected any of these different forms of the bacteria in people with Lyme disease. Even if these round forms were found in human patients, there is no clear evidence that they cause or are in any way associated with chronic Lyme disease. This is all also true for any potential *B. burgdorferi* biofilm formation.

Some of the claims regarding diagnostic tests have some merit. As you will see in the next chapter, blood tests for Lyme disease do suffer from a number of limitations. A major reason many scientists do not believe in chronic Lyme disease is that many of the people who claim they have it don't have a conclusive test showing that they had a prior case of Lyme disease. Although not having a conclusive test does not invalidate the claim of prior Lyme disease, as tests currently used for Lyme disease diagnosis can occasionally be negative both during and long after the initial disease, to claim that these tests don't work is not correct. The performance of these tests has been studied repeatedly to make sure they produce the best results possible. They have been used to correctly diagnose hundreds of thousands of Lyme disease patients over the years. In contrast, many of the alternative tests supported by the chronic Lyme disease groups have not been closely studied, making their usefulness for Lyme disease diagnosis suspect at best.

Some of the claims of coinfections may be reasonable, and the study of coinfections with tick-borne agents is an area that definitely requires more research. However, chronic Lyme disease patients often lack any evidence that they are in fact infected with these other agents. Some of the agents that are claimed to be "coinfecting" agents in chronic Lyme disease have never been shown to be transmitted by ticks, which we will discuss more in Chapter 8. In addition, it has not been shown to be possible for *B. burgdorferi* to be sexually transmitted.

Other individuals that believe they have chronic Lyme disease may in fact have a somewhat similar illness that can be diagnosed, one that is thought to be unrelated to Lyme disease, such as chronic fatigue syndrome or fibromyalgia. A number of patients with neurologic or rheumatologic problems who claim to have chronic Lyme disease ultimately are diagnosed with other illnesses, such as multiple sclerosis, ALS, demyelinating diseases, dementia, rheumatoid arthritis, osteoarthritis, degenerative disease of the spine, and various joint diseases. This means that in all of these cases, a presumptive diagnosis of chronic Lyme disease before exploring other diagnoses was incorrect.

The arguments of chronic Lyme disease advocates that diseases such as autism, Parkinson's disease, multiple sclerosis, or ALS are brought about by Lyme disease are flawed. First, these conditions do not cluster in the northeastern or north-central United States, where Lyme disease is the most common. Second, there is no evidence associating these conditions with a documented past Lyme disease diagnosis.

For these reasons, the concept of chronic Lyme disease as a distinct illness has been rejected by most in the scientific community. This does not mean that scientists believe that the suffering of the people who claim to have this syndrome is not real. It's absolutely clear that many people with chronic Lyme disease do indeed suffer from some very severe and debilitating symptoms, regardless of whether it was actually caused by an infection with *B. burgdorferi*. There is also no doubt that in some of these people, a past infection with *B. burgdorferi* may indeed have been the trigger for some of the current symptoms. What needs to be better understood is: what are the causes in the vast number of individuals where no clear evidence of Lyme disease is found? Sometimes chronic Lyme disease is diagnosed in these individuals simply by exclusion. If there is no clear explanation for your symptoms, for some doctors, Lyme disease can seem to be a likely culprit. However, a diagnosis of chronic Lyme disease can be falsely reassuring and a disservice because you are much less likely to seek an alternative diagnosis and treatment for what might actually be wrong.

Summary

A number of Lyme disease patients continue to have persistent illness long after they finish their antibiotic treatment. When these symptoms continue for longer than six months, this condition is called PTLDS. PTLDS is a subjective disease and the symptoms can vary greatly from patient to patient, making this illness very difficult to properly diagnose. The symptoms mostly include fatigue, muscle aches, headaches, and joint pain, as well as the possibility of a wide range of mental problems. The severity of some of the symptoms can be debilitating, resulting in substantial suffering for people with this condition. PTLDS can greatly affect patients' quality of life, sometimes forcing them to completely change their everyday lifestyle in order to be able live with the disease. To make matters worse, there is also no treatment for this condition.

The causes of PTLDS are not known, although Lyme disease patients who do not get diagnosed early and have more symptoms are more likely to suffer from PTLDS. How often this condition occurs is also not known. Although most scientific literature says that 10 to 20 percent of Lyme disease patients may have persistent symptoms, in some communities, this number may be substantially higher. Because of the uncertainty regarding so many aspects of PTLDS, a condition called "chronic Lyme disease" has gained a large acceptance within communities affected by Lyme disease. Advocates of this condition offer differing explanations for posttreatment symptoms, such as the presence of a persistent infection with *B. burgdorferi*, and as a consequence, they support longer antibiotic treatment. The views of these groups are in disagreement with the standard scientific community on the basis that they lack scientific evidence.

CHAPTER 5

Diagnosing Lyme Disease

E arly diagnosis is crucial for any disease because the quicker you start treatment, the faster you will recover. It is especially important to diagnose Lyme disease early. Obtaining an early diagnosis, followed by a quick start of antibiotic treatment, greatly reduces the chance of developing some of the more severe symptoms of Lyme disease or PTLDS. Your doctor can diagnose Lyme disease in several different ways, depending on how far along you are in the disease. Often, your signs and symptoms will be enough for them to form a diagnosis, and no additional tests will be needed. Other times, they will want to perform tests to confirm that you do, in fact, have the disease. And this is the point where we encounter a substantial divide between the scientific community and the public affected by this disease. Some of the biggest controversies relating to Lyme disease surround the diagnostic tests used to confirm whether or not you have been infected with *B. burgdorferi*. Lyme disease diagnostic tests are complicated, extremely misunderstood, and have several limitations, which leads many patients to believe that they're not reliable. This chapter will explain how the diagnosis of Lyme disease is made and debunk some of the myths about the tests, but also show why some of the concerns regarding them are justified.

Early Recognition

If you find an engorged blacklegged tick embedded in your skin, you need to realize that you may have been exposed to *B. burgdorferi*. There are several things you can and should do at this point. First, remove the tick immediately, using the guidelines outlined in Chapter 2, and save it. You can show it to your doctor, which can help with the diagnosis, or send it away to a laboratory for testing. Then keep an eye on the bite site for the appearance of the EM rash, which will generally appear within three to thirty days after the tick bite. If the rash doesn't appear and you don't develop any symptoms, it means that either the tick was not infected or that it didn't feed for long enough to pass on the infection. If the rash does appear, it means you likely have Lyme disease and you need to go see a doctor as soon as possible.

 Alert

> If you send the tick away for testing, some laboratories may test it quickly and you will know whether you've been exposed within a day or two. It is possible for you to be exposed to *B. burgdorferi* and not get ill. Some people get infected but do not show any symptoms. The reasons for this are unknown.

Finding the Right Doctor

Next, you need to find a doctor. Here is where you may need to do some research. Not all doctors are well informed about Lyme disease. Doctors in areas where Lyme is common tend to be more knowledgeable about the disease because they see it more often and may have even had Lyme disease themselves. This is, of course, a generalization, so even if you live somewhere known to have Lyme disease, you should still do some research and may need to look outside your community.

Finding a well-informed doctor is particularly important for people who suffer from PTLDS. Because this condition is so difficult to diagnose, you need to find a doctor who knows about all of the different symptoms of this condition. How do you find such a doctor? First, ask around in your community. If you live where Lyme disease is more common, there may be a well-regarded doctor who sees Lyme disease patients in your town. If not, there is always the Internet. There are several organizations that educate and help people with Lyme disease, and their websites can offer help in finding a doctor. You can also scan through online support groups and learn about other people's experiences, possibly getting some referrals. You can find the contact information for some of these organizations and support groups in Appendix A: Further Resources.

When searching for a doctor, be aware that there is a wide range of opinions on how to treat Lyme disease. Some of the methods used by different doctors can be controversial. For example, some doctors advocate extended treatment with antibiotics. Most do not. Some may use experimental treatments, which may not be approved by the FDA, even if they are used in countries outside of the United States. If a doctor advises an experimental treatment for your condition, do your homework. Look it up on the Internet, familiarize yourself with it, ask around, perhaps even ask other doctors for their opinion. Learn the pros and cons. Sometimes, experimental treatment can make your condition better. Other times, it can make it worse. Ultimately, you should pick the doctor who is right for you, one you feel is knowledgeable about Lyme disease, and one you can trust.

How Doctors Diagnose Lyme Disease

Doctors can often diagnose Lyme disease based only on the signs and symptoms of the disease, which we went over in Chapter 3, and knowing whether the patient lives in an area where ticks are common. This is especially true if the disease has just begun recently and is in the early localized stage. If it's still early, the diagnostic tests are far less important in obtaining the correct diagnosis than the signs and symptoms themselves.

The appearance of an EM rash is the primary sign that you have Lyme disease. If you live in an area where Lyme disease is common and you show up at your doctor's office with the EM rash, in most cases this will be enough for your doctor to diagnose you with Lyme disease. Remembering if you were bitten by a tick, and even giving it to the doctor to test for *B. burgdorferi*, can be very helpful in the diagnosis. The doctor will ask about your symptoms to learn whether you've had any of the typical flu-like symptoms that come along with the EM rash, and a blood sample may be taken and sent to a specialized laboratory for testing. Although many doctors do this, it is not recommended in very early cases where the rash has just appeared because tests performed this early in the disease often come back negative, even if you do in fact have Lyme disease. We'll discuss why this happens a little later in the chapter. In any case, because the results may not be available for a day or longer, and the presence of the EM rash is the main indicator of Lyme disease anyway, the doctor will likely begin an antibiotic treatment immediately to help clear the infection. You'll learn more about the different antibiotics you may be given in the next chapter.

If you live in an area where blacklegged ticks are not found, and you didn't travel to somewhere Lyme disease is common, but have a rash that could pass for an EM rash, your doctor will very likely consider an alternative diagnosis to Lyme disease. For example, the diagnosis may include any of the diseases that produce a rash that were listed in Chapter 3. Doctors are advised not to test patients for Lyme disease if it's unlikely they came in contact with ticks because this can generate more false positives than true positive results. A false positive would mean a misdiagnosis and improper treatment, including taking some drugs that may not do anything but cause negative side effects without actually curing whatever is actually responsible for the illness you have. For similar reasons, doctors shouldn't test patients who do not have the symptoms of Lyme disease, even if they reside in areas where Lyme disease is common, in order to avoid a possible misdiagnosis and unneeded treatment. For example, if you have a fever, cough, sore throat, and no rash, it's more likely you have the flu, and the doctor shouldn't test you for Lyme disease.

 Alert

> Remember, several different rashes can be mistaken for Lyme disease's characteristic EM rash. In order for it to be diagnosed as an EM rash, the CDC has specified that the rash needs to be at least two inches in diameter.

In some instances, the diagnosis of Lyme disease is not straightforward, especially if some of the typical signs and symptoms are missing. For example, as we mentioned in Chapter 3, not every person with Lyme disease notices the EM rash or even has it in the first place. You may not have any flu-like symptoms either. In these cases, a knowledgeable doctor may recognize other symptoms that could lead to a diagnosis of Lyme disease. You may be asked if you have persistent headaches or shooting pain, which could indicate that you developed Lyme neuroborreliosis. You may be asked if you feel like you have any problems with your heart, which could mean Lyme carditis. The presence or absence of any of these symptoms will be useful for your doctor to ultimately form a diagnosis. However, at this point, where there isn't a clear indicator of Lyme disease, the diagnostic tests become more important in the diagnosis.

Diagnostic Tests

Diagnostic tests are often ordered by a doctor to confirm the diagnosis they made. For instance, if you had a rash that looked like an EM rash, you were likely diagnosed with Lyme disease at the doctor's office, and a positive diagnostic test would later confirm that the initial diagnosis was correct. Other times, these tests will also be ordered when your signs and symptoms are not typical of Lyme disease and there's no obvious diagnosis. Here the results of the tests are required to narrow down the list of what could be causing the symptoms you are having.

Unlike some diagnostic tests that can be performed quickly at the doctor's office, tests for Lyme disease are more complicated and are performed at a specialized laboratory. There are several different types of tests that are typically ordered. Understanding how they work, the pros and cons for each, and why these particular tests are used will hopefully allow you to have a better grasp on the controversy that has been associated with these tests.

Sensitivity and Specificity

All diagnostic tests, regardless of their type, need to fulfill two very important conditions. They need to be *sensitive* and *specific*. The "sensitivity" of a test refers to its ability to detect a pathogen even if it is present only in very small amounts. This is particularly important at the beginning of the disease, where there usually is very little of the pathogen present in your body. Therefore, the more sensitive the test, the more likely it is that it will detect the pathogen and be useful for a diagnosis.

The "specificity" of a test refers to its ability to detect only the pathogen that you are testing for. A Lyme disease test should detect only the infection with *B. burgdorferi*, and not accidentally detect some other bacteria in the sample. For example, if you have the flu and you get tested for Lyme disease with a test that has low specificity, the test may incorrectly detect the influenza virus and show a positive result. However, because the test was for Lyme disease and not the flu, it would appear to be positive for Lyme disease. Scientists call this "cross-reactivity," which means the test is detecting something that it shouldn't and produces a false result.

Diagnostic tests that have cross-reactivity with other bacteria or viruses are highly problematic because they can lead to an incorrect diagnosis and treatments for a disease that is not actually there. The more specific the test, the more likely that the appropriate diagnosis will be achieved. All of the tests currently used for diagnosing Lyme disease have a high degree of both specificity and sensitivity. That does not mean that they are perfect, however. In fact, they have a number of limitations that can affect accurate diagnosis.

ⓔ✔ Fact

Insufficient sensitivity and specificity are the two primary reasons the majority of diagnostic tests that are developed do not get approval to be available to the public.

These days, there are typically two types of tests that are used to diagnose a patient with an infectious disease such as Lyme disease. They are called "molecular" tests and "serologic" tests. In order to better understand Lyme disease diagnosis, you need to know the difference between these tests, as well as the advantages and disadvantages of each.

Molecular Tests

Molecular tests typically use a technique called "polymerase chain reaction," or PCR. The object of PCR is to find the physical presence of the pathogen. It doesn't necessarily find the whole agent; instead, it tests for the presence of some small portion of the pathogen's DNA. Basically, a PCR test increases the amount of DNA of whatever agent it is testing for, and only that agent, so it can be more easily detected. For example, a PCR test for Lyme disease will only amplify *B. burgdorferi* DNA, if it is present. If the bacteria isn't there, nothing will be amplified. Because a healthy person should not have any DNA from *B. burgdorferi* in his or her body, the result of a PCR test for Lyme disease is either a clear yes or no. *B. burgdorferi* will either be detected or not detected. If the test comes back negative, meaning *B. burgdorferi* was not detected, there is no evidence that the person being tested has Lyme disease. If the test is positive, then you have evidence that the person does have the disease.

Serologic Tests

The other type of tests, called "serologic," don't test for whatever is causing the disease directly. Instead, they test for the presence of antibodies fighting against that organism. Once a pathogen infects your body, your immune system responds by producing antibodies to fight back against that agent. Antibodies are proteins that help our immune system recognize and destroy foreign microbes. Antibodies are somewhat specific to each pathogen, meaning antibodies that your body makes to fight off the influenza virus will be different from antibodies for *B. burgdorferi*. Your body makes these antibodies only in response to an infection, which means they wouldn't be in your body if you've never before been infected with that pathogen. For example, if you've never had Lyme disease, you would not have antibodies against *B. burgdorferi*. But once you become infected, your body will begin to make antibodies to *B. burgdorferi*, and serological tests detect their presence. Once the antibodies are made, they can stay in your system for years.

IgM and IgG Antibodies

Your body can produce five different types of antibodies, called IgM, IgG, IgA, IgD, and IgE. Each one is important for different reasons, but the two that are critical for dealing with pathogens such as *B. burgdorferi* are IgM and IgG. When you have Lyme disease, your body produces a huge number of IgM and IgG antibodies that recognize and attack *B. burgdorferi*. However, they are not produced immediately after you get the infection. In fact, it takes several days, perhaps up to a week after the initial infection, before any antibodies to *B. burgdorferi* can be detected. IgM antibodies are the first to be made and, therefore, can be detected first. They usually appear by the time you have a large EM rash and the flu-like symptoms that accompany it. Although IgM antibodies are useful during the initial fight, they are not as good as IgG antibodies. Unfortunately, it takes a while, perhaps a week or so after the appearance of IgM antibodies, for your body to start making IgG antibodies. From this point on, IgG antibodies take over as the main antibodies that your body uses to clear the infection, although some IgM antibodies are still continuously made.

 Fact

Occasionally, production of some antibodies can be harmful to our bodies. Many common allergies are the result of too many antibodies against substances such as dust or pollen.

Because IgM antibodies are produced first, the appearance of only IgM and no IgG antibodies means that you have recently been infected and are still in the early phase of the disease. The detection of IgG antibodies usually means that you have had the infection for several weeks. This difference helps doctors estimate how far along you are in the disease and is crucial for diagnosis.

PCR Tests and Lyme Disease

In many ways, PCR tests are better than serologic tests. They're fairly quick, usually taking just three to five hours after the sample gets to the diagnostic laboratory. PCR is usually very specific as well, meaning the chances of a false positive are low. And a positive PCR result can be treated as conclusive proof that the infectious agent being tested for is actually there. PCR is the best way to achieve a diagnosis for many diseases. However, it is typically not the main test used for Lyme disease. Although it can be very useful in some cases, particularly early in the infection, PCR is much less useful in the later stages of Lyme disease.

When you go to the doctor's office with the signs and symptoms of Lyme disease, the doctor may collect two different types of specimens from you and send them for Lyme disease testing. The majority of the time, a blood sample will be taken. Occasionally, if you have an EM rash, the doctor may also take a small biopsy of your skin directly from the rash site. The specimens can then be sent away for PCR tests.

Blood Testing

As already mentioned, PCR is a specific and sensitive test, so if *B. burgdorferi* is present in the blood, its DNA should be detected. However, the bacteria are not found in the blood throughout the course of the disease. The amount of time *B. burgdorferi* spends in the blood is short, as little as a week or just a few weeks after the initial infection. In addition, even when it is present in the blood, the bacteria are generally found in very low numbers, sometimes so low that they cannot be detected. For a blood sample to be useful for Lyme disease diagnosis, it has to be collected at just the right time, when the bacteria are still present in somewhat high numbers in the blood. In many cases, the blood sample may be collected after the bacteria are already gone from the bloodstream. In these cases, a PCR test will produce a negative result, even though you may in fact have Lyme disease.

Skin Biopsy Testing

Testing a skin biopsy for Lyme disease is much more accurate than testing blood. Because the EM rash results from the bacteria moving through your skin, it's highly likely that there will be bacteria in any biopsy taken from the rash. As a result, testing a skin biopsy is more accurate than testing blood. However, it is still not 100 percent accurate. In some cases, the bacteria may have already left the skin before the sample was taken, even if the rash is still present. Alternatively, even if there still were some bacteria around the rash, simply by unlucky chance the biopsy could have been taken from a spot where the bacteria were not present. A skin biopsy is also a rather invasive procedure, especially for young children, and some parents may have reservations about granting permission. In addition, the presence of the EM rash itself is often enough for a Lyme disease diagnosis. Therefore, a positive PCR result on the EM rash does not really add anything other than confirming the initial diagnosis.

PCR Testing in Later Disease

PCR testing becomes less useful the further along you are in the disease. By the time you move past the early stage, it's difficult to find the bacteria in the skin or blood. At the later stages of Lyme disease, other specimen types are occasionally tested by PCR depending on your symptoms. Cerebrospinal fluid may be taken for a sample if your doctor suspects you are suffering from Lyme neuroborreliosis; a fluid sample from your joints may be taken if your doctor suspects late Lyme disease. Although these tests can help with the diagnosis, neither is very accurate. These PCR tests are frequently negative even if you do have Lyme disease. This is most likely because the bacteria are rarely found in these samples at the time they are taken.

Other Limitations of PCR Testing for Lyme Disease

Another limitation of PCR tests is that because they test for the presence of DNA from the infectious agent, the strain of *B. burgdorferi* that they test for must be the same strain that is causing your illness. If you are infected with a different strain, it may have enough differences in its DNA to cause the tests to come up false negative.

Yet another problem with PCR tests for Lyme disease is that there isn't a single test used by all testing laboratories. PCR tests are not difficult to develop and many testing laboratories each have their own version for Lyme disease. This makes it difficult to identify which tests are the best. A doctor may send your sample to one laboratory where the PCR will be negative. If they send it to another laboratory it may be positive. There may be many reasons for these discrepancies. For example, if a test is not accurate, a false positive result might be caused by cross-reactivity. With so many different tests out there, it's hard to know whether one test is better than another.

The Two-Tiered Test: ELISA and the Western Blot

Right now, most doctors rely on serologic tests for Lyme disease instead of PCR tests. Although many serologic tests have been developed over the years for diagnosing Lyme disease, the only one that the CDC currently recommends is called the two-tiered test. This test was first recommended all the way back in 1995. In the early 1990s, various laboratories were using many different serologic tests for Lyme disease diagnosis, and it turned out that none of them were very accurate. When the tests were compared to one another, a sample that tested positive for *B. burgdorferi* on one test might be negative on another, and vice versa. In order to achieve some level of consistency and accuracy in Lyme disease testing, a new strategy was developed. This strategy involved a two-step process, in which each step consisted of a different type of serologic test.

 Fact

> The recommendation for the use of the two-tiered test was developed by the CDC, along with some other major US agencies, including the US Food and Drug Administration and the National Institutes of Health.

In the two-tiered test for Lyme disease, the results of the first test determine whether the second test will be run. The first step consists of a test called ELISA. If the ELISA test is negative, no further testing is done and the patient is diagnosed as negative. If the ELISA results are positive or borderline positive, an additional test is performed called a Western blot. The two-tiered test is considered positive only if both the ELISA and the Western blot are positive.

 Fact

> ELISA stands for enzyme-linked immunosorbent assay. The ELISA test is probably the most common serologic test used today, not just for Lyme disease but for a wide range of infectious diseases.

Lyme ELISA

The first of the two-tiered tests is the ELISA. In this test, over a thousand proteins that are present in a single strain of *B. burgdorferi* are stuck to the bottom of a small plastic plate. When a blood sample arrives at the lab, it is separated into two parts. One part contains just the blood cells and doesn't get tested. The other part, which is tested, is the liquid, called the serum, which has all of the antibodies in it. During the ELISA, a small portion of the serum is added to the plate that has the *B. burgdorferi* proteins. If antibodies to *B. burgdorferi* are in the serum, they will attach to the proteins, just like they would normally do if they were attacking the bacteria in the body. In a positive ELISA test, when the antibodies attach, there is a color change from clear to yellow. If the test is negative, there will be no color change and the plate will stay a clear color. Even if positive, however, the results of the ELISA test alone are not reported until the Western blot test is performed.

ⓔ✔ Fact

In a serologic test such as an ELISA, an "equivocal" result can sometimes be obtained. Equivocal is a borderline positive result that isn't really a positive or a negative. This could be caused by a range of results that overlap between a small portion of Lyme disease patients and a small portion of healthy individuals. Because it's not considered positive, it requires further examination with other tests such as the Western blot.

The Western Blot Test

The second part of the two-tiered test for Lyme disease is a Western blot, which is always run following a positive ELISA to confirm the result. The Western blot can help clarify equivocal results on the ELISA as well as identify any samples that were falsely positive.

In the two-tiered test, there are two types of Western blot tests that are performed: an IgM Western blot and an IgG Western blot. The IgM Western blot, as you would expect from the name, is used only to test for the presence of IgM antibodies found in the early stages of the disease. The IgG Western blot only tests for IgG antibodies that are made later in the disease and identifies the disease in the early disseminated and late Lyme disease stages.

Proteins from the same strain of *B. burgdorferi* that were used in the ELISA are used for this test. The test starts by using electricity to first separate all the proteins from each other by their size and then make them stick to a special type of paper. When the serum from the sample is added, any antibodies against *B. burgdorferi* that are present will attach themselves to the proteins. Just like in the ELISA, there is a color change when the antibodies attach to the proteins. Because the *B. burgdorferi* proteins are separated by size, multiple colored bands will appear. For example, if a person has antibodies to ten different proteins from *B. burgdorferi*, they will likely appear as ten different bands on the Western blot.

 Fact

Although only three IgM and ten IgG bands are scored in Lyme disease Western blots, this does not mean that these are the only bands present. Often other bands will appear, but they can be highly variable from patient to patient, so scientists usually just ignore them for scoring purposes.

The number of bands that appear in Western blot tests for Lyme disease is what determines whether the tests are positive or negative, with each type of Western blot requiring a different amount. Scientists studied many samples from positive Lyme disease specimens across the United States and figured out that in an IgM Western blot, three bands are important for diagnosis. Not everyone with Lyme disease will have antibodies that will produce all three bands. On the other hand, even when healthy people are tested, they can frequently produce one band because of cross-reactivity. Therefore, at least two of the three bands on an IgM Western blot need to appear for it to be considered positive.

For the IgG Western blot, ten different bands are frequently seen in Lyme disease–positive patients. Just like with the IgM Western blot, not everyone will have all of the bands appear, and samples from people without Lyme disease can occasionally show one or two bands. Therefore, for a Lyme disease IgG Western blot test to be considered positive, at least five bands must appear.

Why Are ELISAs and Western Blots Linked?

The need to run two tests has been somewhat confusing to the public in the past. There are a number of reasons why the two-tiered test is structured the way it is. First of all, the two tests that comprise the two-tiered test are not independent of each other. In fact, they are both similar in that they typically use the same strain of *B. burgdorferi* as a target, and one test should not "work better" than the other. In some ways, they are one test done in two different ways. The main difference is that the ELISA detects all of the IgM and IgG antibodies that recognize and attach to every single *B. burgdorferi* protein. This can sometimes include antibodies made to fight against other infectious agents, that, because of cross-reactivity, will incorrectly attach to one of the *B. burgdorferi* proteins. This means that there's a greater chance for a false positive on the ELISA. This can be corrected with the Western blot test because scientists can look at just a few specific proteins, making the test more specific than an ELISA.

So why don't we just use the Western blot test and ignore the ELISA altogether? Unfortunately, the Western blot tests, especially the IgM Western blots, can be rather subjective. The person running the test could easily score a band wrong, calling it positive when it should be negative or vice versa, and accidentally create a misdiagnosis. Running the ELISA first makes it so there's at least a chance that *B. burgdorferi* antibodies are present in the sample. These two tests, individually, are not perfect, but together they work as great checks against each other and combine to make an accurate test for Lyme disease.

 Fact

In the Western blot part of the two-tiered test for Lyme disease, both IgM and IgG tests are run unless the doctor knows for a fact that the patient has had symptoms for more than thirty days. In this case, only the IgG Western blot test is run. IgM Western blot tests run on samples from patients who have had the disease for more than a month create some very confusing results that are difficult to score properly.

Controversies Around the Two-Tiered Test

One of the biggest controversies in the field of Lyme disease is the use of the two-tiered test as the main recommended diagnostic test. According to the CDC, when performed and interpreted in accordance with the existing guidelines, the two-tiered testing is very useful for diagnosis in the two later stages of Lyme disease: the early disseminated and late Lyme disease. It's been shown to accurately diagnose between 70 and 80 percent of people in the early disseminated stage and is nearly 100 percent accurate for people in the late Lyme disease stage.

The biggest problem of the two-tiered test is that it is not useful for the early localized stage. Unfortunately, this is when accurate tests are required the most. The vast majority of Lyme disease specimens that are sent by doctors for testing are from this stage, and an accurate diagnosis is critical in order to stop the development of more severe symptoms and PTLDS. In most cases, at the time the blood is drawn, the immune system hasn't made enough antibodies to *B. burgdorferi* for them to be detected by the test. Studies have shown that only about 40 percent of samples from patients with early localized Lyme disease are accurately diagnosed with the two-tiered test. When testing patients within the first week of the disease, less than 15 percent have come back positive. For this reason, testing blood collected very early in the course of the disease, such as immediately after you remove the tick or after noticing the EM rash, is not recommended by the CDC. The majority of the time, these tests will come back negative and not be useful, even if you are infected. In these cases, doctors should base their diagnosis on the presence of the EM rash.

Even if you did have a test early on in the disease and it came back negative, you can go back in a few weeks later for a second sample to be taken. By that time, typically two to four weeks after the first sample, you should have produced enough antibodies to be detected by the tests.

Occasionally, even this follow-up sample comes back negative. A negative result on both samples is more difficult to clarify. In most people, these repeated negative results are presumed to be the result of the treatment clearing the infection before the body can develop enough antibodies for the test to detect. This can be especially difficult for patients with PTLDS. Because documented evidence of prior Lyme disease is required for a PTLDS diagnosis, patients with actual PTLDS but with two negative tests may be misdiagnosed and treated for some other illness.

ⓔ✔ Fact

The frequency of Lyme disease patients who test negative both before and after treatment is believed to be very low. However, in one study, it was shown to be as high as 39 percent.

This can also make it difficult for patients who don't have all of the signs and symptoms, such as those who don't have an obvious EM rash. Because they don't have the stereotypical symptoms for a doctor to diagnose the disease that way and the tests come back negative, the treatment could be delayed, and the risk of developing late Lyme disease or PTLDS greatly increases.

Even when the two-tiered test does diagnose early disease, these tests may not be fully accurate. A major problem with IgM Western blots is that they frequently produce false-positive results. IgM antibodies are not as exact as IgG and are "sticky," meaning they can often bind to wrong targets. IgM antibodies in your blood that were made to protect against other pathogens can often cross-react and attach to *B. burgdorferi* proteins. One study showed that up to 29 percent of "positive" IgM Western blots were actually false positives, and approximately 5 percent of all IgM Western blot tests generate false-positive results, even when testing healthy individuals. Therefore, IgM Western blots are clearly not the most specific tests of early infection.

Another well-known problem with the two-tiered test is the subjectivity associated with the scoring of the Western blot test. Analyzing the bands and deciding whether they're positive or negative is typically done by the laboratory staff. Interpretation of the bands may be confusing—a borderline positive band to one person may simply be negative to another. These days, labs will usually have several staff members score the bands to reduce this subjectivity, and in some the scoring is now automated using computer software.

✅ Fact

A large number of samples are tested for Lyme disease each year. A study by the CDC estimated that roughly 3.4 million samples were tested in 2008, at an estimated cost of $492 million, the majority of which were two-tiered tests.

Following the initial infection, antibodies to *B. burgdorferi* stick around for years. Because the diagnosis with the two-tiered test is based on whether there are any antibodies against *B. burgdorferi*, it is difficult to separate a reinfection from an older infection. This is also why a serologic test cannot be used as proof that the infection was cured, since serologic tests will continue to be positive indefinitely.

Although the two-tiered test does have major advantages, such as its success in identifying Lyme disease in its later two stages, it obviously has significant problems as well, which has led to some major criticisms by patients who identify themselves as suffering from "chronic Lyme disease." As we discussed in Chapter 4, many of these people have never been officially diagnosed with Lyme disease. One reason many of these people say they were never diagnosed is because these tests simply missed them, even if they actually had Lyme disease. Until we get a more effective test, these concerns will naturally remain.

Other Tests

Because of the limitations of the two-tiered and PCR tests, many research labs have begun to develop alternative tests for Lyme disease. A number of different groups are currently testing numerous molecular, serologic (both ELISA and non–ELISA-based), and even biochemical tests for better ways to diagnose Lyme disease. Most, if not all, of these tests claim to be an improvement over the two-tiered test. The ultimate goal is to potentially replace and eventually eliminate the two-tiered test with these newer, better tests.

C6 ELISA

Because the standard ELISA used in the two-tiered tests can occasionally produce false-positive results, researchers have spent a lot of time and effort trying to develop other ELISAs, ones that are more specific to *B. burgdorferi* and limit cross-reactivity. One way to make ELISAs more specific to *B. burgdorferi* is to use fewer *B.*

burgdorferi proteins as targets for antibodies. That may seem counterintuitive, but using only a few proteins that are unique to *B. burgdorferi* and removing the kinds of proteins that other bacteria have should reduce cross-reactivity.

Based on this idea, many different Lyme disease ELISA tests have been developed over the years, with varying degrees of success when tested on human specimens. However, there is one ELISA that has been very useful for diagnosis. It is based on a protein called VlsE. Researchers have found that all patients with Lyme disease seem to make a large number of antibodies against one specific fragment of VlsE, called the C6 region. This fragment is present in every single strain of *B. burgdorferi* as well as *B. garinii* and *B. afzelii*, the bacteria that cause Lyme disease in Europe. Also, it doesn't appear in any other bacteria, so it is very specific for Lyme disease. By using just this small C6 fragment as the target, scientists were able to produce an ELISA test for Lyme disease that was more specific than the standard ELISA. This test is called the C6 ELISA to differentiate it from other ELISA tests.

Without a secondary test such as a Western blot, the C6 ELISA is actually more sensitive than the two-tiered test for diagnosing early Lyme disease. However, it is not as accurate as the standard ELISA and the Western blot combined. Because of this, it is not used as a single test for Lyme disease. That being said, it has been recommended that testing laboratories should use it as part of the two-tiered test instead of the Western blot. There, the C6 ELISA would perform a similar function to the Western blots in confirming the original ELISA but wouldn't have the same subjectivity problem as the Western blots. In addition, the combination of a standard ELISA coupled with the C6 ELISA would make the two-tiered test more sensitive and increase the chance of detecting early Lyme disease.

Culture

The best way to test for any disease would be to grow the bacteria in the laboratory from a sample taken from you when you were sick. Any pathogen can be easily identified when it is growing in culture. A positive culture, where the microbe is alive and actively dividing, provides 100 percent certain evidence that the bacteria was present in the original sample and therefore provides an irrefutable diagnosis. In the early days of Lyme disease testing, this was a common method for obtaining a definitive diagnosis. It's still occasionally used today, particularly to confirm a previously made diagnosis. However, it is highly impractical for the majority of infectious diseases, including Lyme disease, where you need a quick diagnosis. A bacterial or viral culture may take days, or in the case of Lyme disease, weeks, to produce enough microorganisms that can be detected. In addition, *B. burgdorferi* sometimes cannot be cultured even in patients with all the signs and symptoms of Lyme disease. Because of all of these problems with cultures, other means of detection are used for quick and accurate diagnosis.

Next-Generation Sequencing

In the past decade, a new molecular test, called either next-generation sequencing or high-throughput sequencing, has become much more common across the entire molecular biology field. It basically combines the PCR tests we talked about earlier with DNA sequencing. During next-generation sequencing, instead of increasing just the DNA of the agent you're looking for, the amount of every single piece of DNA in the sample is increased, then scientists identify everything. This is incredibly useful for diagnostics. Because everything is amplified, the test is not biased to look for any one particular pathogen, and strain differences of *B. burgdorferi* do not matter. Different groups have started to use this as an alternative means to PCR diagnosis.

Metabolomics

Instead of looking at DNA and antibodies, some groups have started to try and identify changes in your metabolism that occur from a *B. burgdorferi* infection. These types of studies are called "metabolomics." So far, forty-four biochemical differences have been identified between people with early Lyme disease and people without. These changes happen soon after infection, much earlier than the time it takes for antibodies to *B. burgdorferi* to appear. Although it's still early in the research, these changes could potentially be used to diagnose early Lyme disease and have been shown, in preliminary comparisons, to be substantially more accurate than two-tiered testing in early Lyme disease.

Microscopy

You may wonder why scientists even have to run all of these tests. Why can't they just take a drop of blood, look at it under a microscope, and see the bacteria swimming around? After all, that's how a lot of other infectious diseases are diagnosed. Unfortunately, it's not that easy with Lyme disease, for the same reasons PCR tests often fail. The bacteria simply might not be in the blood, and even if they are, they may be so scarce that chances are you will not see them anyway. And because they are so rare, anything that accidentally slips in while the sample is being prepared, such as a piece of hair or dust (trust me, it does happen), may get misidentified as a spirochete and result in you getting misdiagnosed.

Difficulty in Test Development

Despite these promising results, high costs and the difficulty of implementing many of these newer tests in a standard laboratory are major limitations. The cost for most of these tests to examine a single sample is currently much higher than the cost of a typical two-tiered test. Many of these tests also require special equipment that is not available in most laboratories. It is expected, however, that as testing continues and these tests are proven to be more effective, these issues can be fixed and many of these tests can be made available to the public.

In addition, a number of laboratories have developed their own in-house tests for Lyme disease that they offer to patients on a per-fee basis as an alternative to the two-tiered test. The accuracy and usefulness of many of these tests have not been verified, and therefore they are not reliable ways to diagnose Lyme disease, but they are available if you search for them.

Whether any of the in-house tests are better than the two-tiered test remains unclear. However, what is clear is that there needs to be an improvement in Lyme disease diagnosis over the two-tiered test. Better tests are desperately needed; however, they need to be critically evaluated and show clear improvement in performance over current tests prior to being available to the public.

Summary

Lyme disease can be diagnosed in two different ways. Early in the disease, it is usually diagnosed based on characteristic signs and symptoms, especially the EM rash, and no other tests are necessary. For patients where clear signs and symptoms are absent, diagnostic tests become much more important. The two main types of diagnostic tests are molecular, which look for the DNA of *B. burgdorferi* in a sample, or serologic, which look for the presence of antibodies to this bacteria. These tests need to be specific to *B. burgdorferi* and sensitive enough to be able to detect the bacteria even when there aren't many to be found. The primary molecular test is PCR, which can be used early in the disease but can often be negative when blood is tested because of the lack of bacteria in the sample. PCR tests become less useful later on and are often negative even in patients with active disease.

Serologic tests are more useful in the disseminated and late Lyme disease stages. The serologic test used for Lyme disease diagnosis is called the two-tiered test and consists of an ELISA followed by two Western blots, one testing for IgM antibodies and the other for IgG antibodies. Although it has many positives, the two-tiered test also has several limitations that have led to major criticism regarding its use. It is not helpful in the early stages of the infection, which is when most patients are tested. It is also very subjective, can often be false positive, and can produce negative results even in patients with known Lyme disease. Because of these problems, many other tests have been developed with the goal of replacing the two-tiered test as the primary test for Lyme disease. One such test, the C6 ELISA, has already been adapted by many laboratories as a substitute for the Western blot. Other tests show promise for use in the future, but problems with costs and implementation may limit their use. There are also other tests that are already being used in some laboratories, but at this time it is not clear whether they are an improvement over the two-tiered test.

CHAPTER 6

Treatment for Lyme Disease

et's say you've been diagnosed with Lyme disease. Your doctor will then prescribe you antibiotics to help you fight off the infection. The doctor will also tell you that antibiotic treatment is very effective in most people and you should get well fairly soon. However, as you start your treatment, you may be a little nervous. You may have heard that treating Lyme disease is extremely difficult. You also may have heard that you can't get rid of the infection completely and may require multiple doses of antibiotics over the next few months. Many people, unfortunately, have this rather incorrect perception of Lyme disease treatment. In this chapter, you will read all about how Lyme disease is treated, how long the treatments last, and some treatments to avoid.

Antibiotics

Most people know that antibiotics are drugs used to treat diseases but that's a little too broad a definition. Antibiotics are the standard drug prescribed by doctors to treat any infection that is caused by bacteria. The majority of antibiotics come from natural sources, usually a fungus or bacteria, that can prevent the growth of other microbes. When scientists discover such a substance, they purify it and try to make it into a drug. Generally, the antibiotics that you use now have been modified by scientists from their original form to make them even more effective.

Several different types of antibiotics are typically prescribed, but they all work in one of two ways: they are either bactericidal or bacteriostatic. A bactericidal antibiotic kills the bacteria, whereas a bacteriostatic antibiotic will only stop them from multiplying, letting your immune system do the rest. Antibiotics are specific for the type of bacteria that are causing your symptoms, which is why a certain antibiotic will be prescribed to treat Lyme disease, while a different one may be given for an ear infection. Taking a wrong antibiotic to treat Lyme disease may have little to no effect. Antibiotics that are specific to a group of bacteria are called narrow-spectrum antibiotics, while ones that can be used against a wide range of bacteria are called broad-spectrum antibiotics.

🅔✓ Fact

Penicillin was the first antibiotic. It was discovered in 1928 by the Scottish physician and scientist Alexander Fleming. He determined that a particular fungus, called *Penicillium*, produced a substance that could prevent bacteria from growing around it. Other scientists later realized that by purifying the substance, it could be used to fight off infections in people. The antibiotic was first used in the early 1940s and was given the name penicillin, after the fungus that it originated from.

How Do Antibiotics Work?

The main goal of an antibiotic is to stop harmful bacteria from dividing within your body. The less harmful bacteria, the fewer symptoms you will likely have, and the easier it will be for your immune system to destroy it. Many people think that antibiotics are the only thing that stops a bacterial infection. They certainly help, but your immune system also has to do a lot of the work. Antibiotics and your immune system work together to get rid of the pathogenic bacteria. This is why bacteriostatic antibiotics, which don't kill bacteria, are still useful. They ensure that no additional bacteria will arise, leaving your immune system to take care of the rest.

How they do it can vary depending on their type, but all antibiotics prevent bacteria from performing some important function that keeps them alive. For example, bacteria have a structure around them called a "cell wall." It is a very important structure that bacteria need for survival. Some antibiotics such as penicillin (and any others that end with -cillin) prevent them from making that wall, killing the bacteria. Other antibiotics prevent bacteria from making proteins, which every cell needs to live.

❓ Question

Why don't antibiotics harm our cells?
The reason antibiotics are so useful is that they specifically target bacterial cells and not human cells. The structure of a bacterial cell is quite different from that of a human cell. The parts that antibiotics target are unique to bacteria, so antibiotics have no effect on human cells.

Oral and Intravenous Antibiotics

If you have a bacterial infection, you can be treated with antibiotics in two ways. The most common way to take antibiotics is through a pill or liquid that you swallow, known as oral antibiotics. If the bacterial infection is particularly severe and needs stronger treatment, intravenous (IV) antibiotics are used. IV antibiotics have several advantages over their oral counterparts if immediate strong treatment is required. They're injected directly into your bloodstream, which allows them to reach the site of the infection much more quickly because they don't have to go through your digestive system. IV antibiotics can also be given in higher doses than oral antibiotics. Once the IV is inserted into your vein, it usually takes as little as half an hour for the drugs to start working.

Side Effects of Antibiotics

Antibiotics are drugs, and like any drugs, they can result in some side effects. The most common side effects usually affect the digestive system. Antibiotics, especially broad-spectrum antibiotics, cause large changes in the bacteria found in your gastrointestinal tract. Billions of bacteria live inside your intestines and a large portion of them (sometimes called the "good bacteria") have a positive effect on your overall health. These bacteria prevent other potentially pathogenic bacteria from establishing an infection and causing disease. They also help your immune system to function properly. Treatment with antibiotics not only kills the infecting microbe, but kills a great number of these good bacteria as well. This can cause the side effects that sometimes occur with antibiotic treatment, including stomach pain, bloating, vomiting, loss of appetite, and mild to severe diarrhea. These symptoms usually go away once you finish the treatment. In addition, because you wipe out the "good" bacteria, other pathogens can sometimes take their place, causing problems such as yeast infections and diarrheal disease.

Some people can also have allergic reactions to antibiotics, including several antibiotics that are usually prescribed for Lyme disease. A typical allergic reaction to an antibiotic will include a rash, some wheezing and coughing, and difficulty breathing due to tightness in your throat. If any of these symptoms appear after taking an antibiotic, tell your doctor right away.

If your antibiotics are administered through an IV rather than a pill, you may experience some other side effects. One of the most serious is an infection with another, antibiotic-resistant bacteria living in the IV line. These infections can result in severe, even fatal, disease.

 Fact

All of the billions of microorganisms found in your body are called your "microbiome." You can have very different microbiomes in different parts of your body. For instance, the types of bacteria that live in your intestines are very different from the bacteria that live on your skin. All of your various microbiomes interacting together in harmony is very important to your health.

Recommended Treatment for Lyme Disease

Antibiotics are the standard treatment for Lyme disease. In general, the sooner you begin an antibiotic treatment, the quicker your symptoms will begin to disappear. Early treatment also helps prevent the development of additional symptoms and lessens the likelihood of persistent symptoms. Several first-line antibiotics are typically prescribed for Lyme disease, depending on the stage and the severity of the disease.

 Fact

First-line antibiotics are the antibiotics that will be prescribed first, because they are likely to be most effective on whatever infection they are prescribed for.

Early Lyme Disease Treatment

For the treatment of Lyme disease when the EM rash appears, you'll most often be prescribed an antibiotic called doxycycline. Some other common antibiotics at this stage include amoxicillin and cefuroxime axetil. In rarer cases, usually only if you have allergies to these other drugs, you might be given azithromycin. It's not a first-line drug because sometimes it's not as effective for Lyme disease as the other drugs used. The following is a summary of the antibiotics prescribed for treatment of early Lyme disease, including the dosage and duration of the treatment:

- **Doxycycline**—100 milligram (mg) pill taken twice daily for ten days to three weeks
- **Amoxicillin**—500 mg pill taken three times daily for two to three weeks
- **Cefuroxime axetil**—500 mg pill taken twice daily for two to three weeks
- **Azithromycin**—500 mg pill taken once daily for seven to ten days

If you have Lyme disease, you will only be given one of these antibiotics for treatment. Do not mix any of these drugs because they are not meant to be taken in any combination with one another. Taking them together may actually reduce their effectiveness.

Which antibiotic to prescribe and how long you need to take them is ultimately the doctor's decision and can vary depending on the patient. For example, children may be treated differently than adults. The best length of treatment can, of course, be different for every patient. In the past, three weeks of antibiotics was generally recommended for just about every patient with early Lyme disease. However, recent research has shown that a shorter ten-day doxycycline treatment is just as effective as the three-week treatment and can now be recommended instead of the longer therapy. How long the treatment should last can vary from doctor to doctor, depending on their past experience in treating patients with Lyme disease.

The EM rash will usually resolve within a few days or weeks after you start the treatment. The other symptoms of early Lyme disease, such as the headache, muscle pain, or fatigue, may take longer, but should get better and better over the next few months. In the United States, anywhere between 70 and more than 90 percent of Lyme disease patients treated with antibiotics will return to their normal health by the end of the first year.

Front-Line Early Lyme Disease Antibiotics

Each of the front-line antibiotics is effective for treating Lyme disease, but each of them is also slightly different. Because it's always good to know what you're putting into your body, especially when it comes to drugs, here's a quick rundown on each of the three front-line antibiotics.

Doxycycline is a broad-spectrum bacteriostatic antibiotic. It works by stopping *B. burgdorferi* from making proteins. It's used to treat a wide variety of infections, including intestinal infections, eye infections, gum disease, and more. You'll get the side effects typical of other antibiotics with doxycycline, mostly gastrointestinal problems, with the exception that sun exposure can lead to a higher likelihood of a rash. Unless the condition is life threatening, it is not recommended for children under eight or pregnant women.

Amoxicillin is a bactericidal antibiotic that is basically penicillin that has been modified in a lab. If you're allergic to penicillin, you shouldn't take this drug. Because it's made from penicillin, anyone allergic to penicillin will also be allergic to amoxicillin. Amoxicillin is a broad-spectrum antibiotic that prevents bacteria from making the cell wall. Besides Lyme disease, amoxicillin is used to treat infections of the ear, skin, urinary tract, and respiratory tract.

The side effects are the same as for any other antibiotic, with rash and nausea being the most common.

Cefuroxime axetil is a bactericidal antibiotic that works similarly to amoxicillin, preventing the bacteria from producing the cell wall. Other than Lyme disease, it's used to treat infections of the ear, heart, skin, bone, joint, and urinary tract, as well as meningitis and more. The most common side effect of cefuroxime axetil is diarrhea.

Azithromycin is a bacteriostatic antibiotic that prevents bacteria from making proteins. In addition to Lyme disease, azithromycin is prescribed against ear and skin infections, strep throat, pneumonia, gastrointestinal infections, and sexually transmitted infections such as gonorrhea and chlamydia. The most common side effect of azithromycin is diarrhea.

❉ Essential

Most antibiotics have two names listed on the package. One is the capitalized brand name that is created by the pharmaceutical company, and the other is a generic name of the antibiotic. For example, Zithromax is the brand name for azithromycin.

Treatment for Early Disseminated Lyme Disease and Late Lyme Disease

If you develop Lyme neuroborreliosis or Lyme carditis, your treatment may vary depending on how severe your symptoms become. If your symptoms aren't as bad and you don't have to be hospitalized, you may be given the same oral antibiotics you would for the early stage, with the treatment lasting for two to three weeks. However, severe symptoms mean you'll have to be admitted to the hospital and treated with IV antibiotics. The IV antibiotic typically used for Lyme disease treatment is ceftriaxone, which is generally given once daily for two weeks. If at any point your symptoms begin to go away and you're allowed to leave the hospital, you can finish the required two-week treatment with any of the first-line oral antibiotics prescribed by your doctor. You could also continue the IV treatment at home with the help of a visiting physician's assistant.

If the Lyme disease has progressed to the arthritis stage, the treatment is the same as for the early stage, except you'll have to take the antibiotics for four weeks instead of ten days or so. If your symptoms still don't stop, you will either be given another four-week dose of oral antibiotics or they'll switch you over to ceftriaxone, twice daily for up to four weeks. If you continue to have arthritis after both treatments, you may be diagnosed with antibiotic-refractory Lyme arthritis, which we talked about in Chapter 3. In this case, further antibiotic treatment is not recommended, as it's been shown not to work, especially if tests indicate no presence of any *B. burgdorferi* in your joints. Instead, you'll likely be given some anti-inflammatory drugs, antirheumatic drugs, or injections of corticosteroids to help with your symptoms.

 Fact

Ceftriaxone is an antibiotic used for treatment of Lyme disease and many other infections. Because, unlike other drugs prescribed for Lyme disease, it is administered by IV, pain at the site of the needle insertion is a common side effect.

People with facial palsy recover very quickly after treatment begins. People with radicular pain and meningitis take a little bit longer, improving within days to weeks. However, in some cases, the nerves may have been injured permanently and they can't be completely recovered. Patients with late neuroborreliosis have a much more gradual improvement of their symptoms, usually starting a few months after the treatment finishes and continuing slowly for up to one to two years. Patients who get Lyme carditis have an excellent outcome following treatment, with symptoms typically disappearing after one to six weeks. If a patient suffers from severe heart block, the improvement to a mild block or normal heartbeat should take about six days. Lyme arthritis may take longer to subside, anywhere from several weeks to a few months.

Selecting the Optimal Antibiotics

There are several ways to choose the best antibiotics for treating a particular disease. Usually, scientists select commonly used antibiotics and examine how these drugs work on patients who have the disease they are studying. The first such tests of antibiotics for Lyme disease were performed in 1980 and 1981, and showed that the antibiotics penicillin and tetracycline worked well against *B. burgdorferi* infections. Further studies over the years found other antibiotics that now make up the list of first-line drugs for Lyme disease. However, it is not practical to test a wide array of different drugs on patients. Instead, scientists can learn a lot about how useful a drug may be by first testing it in the laboratory. The bacteria are grown in multiple different cultures and then a different antibiotic is added to each one. The scientists study the growth of the bacteria over the next few days to see how each treatment affects it. The antibiotics that are best at stopping the growth of the bacteria are the ones that are then selected for clinical trials on patients. This is how scientists learned that azithromycin may be very useful, since it prevented growth of *B. burgdorferi* in culture.

Antibiotic Treatment after a Tick Bite

If you removed an engorged tick, you may be tempted to start antibiotic treatment immediately, on the off chance that the tick that bit you was infected. Could it be helpful? At least one study showed that it could be. Taking a single 200 mg dose of doxycycline (prescribed by your doctor) within seventy-two hours after removal of a blacklegged tick will reduce the chances of you getting Lyme disease. However, because antibiotic treatment for every single tick bite is not reasonable, this way of preventing Lyme disease is not generally recommended. On some occasions, it is allowed and your doctor will prescribe you the antibiotic, provided the following conditions are met:

1. You live in an area where at least one out of five ticks are infected.
2. You can prove conclusively that a blacklegged tick was attached for more than thirty-six hours.
3. The treatment can be given within seventy-two hours after removing the tick.

Appropriate Length of Treatment

The question of how long treatments for Lyme disease should last is a matter of some debate in the Lyme disease community. Not everyone responds the same way to antibiotics, and neither do the strains of *B. burgdorferi*. The treatments we've talked about in this chapter are the generally accepted guidelines based on established research and doctors' experiences, and are most likely what your doctor is going to prescribe. However, they may not be right for everyone. For some patients, the first treatment fails, they continue to get worse, and they need to be put on other antibiotics. As we've talked about before, not all doctors agree with the current recommendations. Some doctors believe that the recommended length is not effective enough and that to truly work, the treatment needs to be longer.

As mentioned in previous chapters, a significant number of people with Lyme disease end up having symptoms that continue after the treatments end. If you completed your treatment but continue to have persistent symptoms, it makes sense to think that perhaps the antibiotics didn't fully work. Maybe not all of the bacteria in your body have been eliminated and maybe another antibiotic regimen will kill the remaining bacteria. A small group of doctors, typically associated with the movement that advocates for the concept of "chronic Lyme disease," think along the same lines. These doctors say that *B. burgdorferi* can hide in places within your body that antibiotics can't get enough access to in order to completely eliminate the disease, and that only continuous treatment can ensure that your symptoms will eventually go away.

However, the group of doctors known as the Infectious Diseases Society of America (IDSA), who set the recommended treatment for Lyme disease, disagree and think this extended antibiotic treatment has absolutely no positive effects on the treatment of Lyme disease. These two opposing views have been the subject of much intense debate and controversy in the Lyme community for many years. Let's take a look at this argument more closely because it is very important for everyone to know all the facts about this contentious issue. First, let's examine why continual antibiotic treatment is not a trivial thing.

Studying Long-Term Treatments of Lyme Disease

A substantial part of the argument about prolonged antibiotic treatment is the risk versus reward of additional treatment. Three clinical studies in the United States and one in Europe have examined the effectiveness of prolonged antibiotic treatment for PTLDS. The results of these studies all argue against long-term antibiotic treatment. In two of the four studies, a small amount of improvement was seen, while in the other two, no improvement was seen at all. On the other hand, side effects of treatment were common in all of the studies, including blood clots, severe allergic infections, and new infections from the IV treatments. Even in the two studies that did show improvement, the risks were too high to justify the continued treatment. Although nobody died in those four studies, there have been at least two documented deaths of patients from bacterial infections that resulted from long-term IV antibiotic therapy for Lyme disease.

Antibiotic treatments are necessary to treat Lyme disease. However, if there is no evidence that the treatment will work, especially when the person may not have had the disease in the first place, continuous treatments will not only not provide any benefit, but will also increase the risk of some very serious side effects.

Many in the community who promote long-term antibiotic treatment disagree with the conclusions of these studies. They claim that the studies did not include enough patients in order to clearly see whether there was any improvement, and point to the fact that some improvement was actually seen in two of the studies. This argument for continued antibiotic treatment centers around the possibility that live *B. burgdorferi* bacteria are still present in the body and that these are what cause the symptoms in patients with PTLDS or chronic Lyme disease. This scenario has never been disproven and may indeed account for some of these symptoms. Prolonged antibiotic treatment will continue to be a controversial topic until there is a clearer answer to this question. Unfortunately, we are not there yet.

Resistance to Antibiotics

One of the major problems with widespread use of antibiotics is the emergence of antibiotic-resistant bacteria. Infections with these bacteria are incredibly difficult to treat, and can require costly and occasionally toxic alternative drugs. Can *B. burgdorferi* become antibiotic resistant? Luckily, the answer appears to be no. In over forty years of research into this bacteria, there have been no reports of any strains of *B. burgdorferi* becoming antibiotic resistant. Even when scientists were trying to create antibiotic-resistant strains in a lab, they couldn't. Therefore, it seems that resistance to antibiotics is one thing that you don't have to worry about.

🔘 Alert

Long-term use of antibiotics has given rise to the emergence of drug resistance in bacteria. By using antibiotics, we are killing the bacteria that are susceptible to the drug, but there is always some small amount of bacteria that are naturally resistant. While the other non-resistant bacteria die, these resistant bacteria will continue to divide until they become the dominant population. Using antibiotics when they are not needed provides a better chance for bacteria to adapt to these drugs, and contributes to this major developing health problem.

Complementary and Alternative Approaches

If you suffer from persistent symptoms following Lyme disease treatment you may be unpleasantly surprised to find that you have limited options to help you deal with your condition. At this point, you might start considering other remedies to help reduce your symptoms. Some of these may be questionable therapies that you should approach with skepticism, which we talk about a little later in the chapter. Others may be holistic therapies that have been practiced for centuries and have increasingly grown in acceptance in Western cultures. What are these therapies and can they actually help in alleviating symptoms of Lyme disease?

Antibiotic treatments are the only recommended therapy that has been shown to be effective in people with this disease. Although some people who are mistrustful of doctors and pharmaceuticals may be tempted to use only alternative treatments, this is not recommended, mainly based on the lack of credible evidence that they can provide relief and cure the infection. More important, by not adequately treating the infection early, you may be leaving yourself vulnerable to the development of additional, more severe symptoms of the disease.

What, then, can you do when your initial antibiotic treatment was not fully effective? What if you continue to have pain, feel disoriented, or are constantly tired? Do you continue your treatment with more antibiotics? Some doctors may suggest doing so. However, such treatment may not have any additional benefits, and you can face some serious side effects. If you decide that continued antibiotic treatment is not something you want to pursue, there is not much more that traditional medicine can offer. At this point, some people do try alternative, natural treatments in the hope that they can alleviate some pain. The use of these therapies will ultimately be your decision because some doctors may not recommend them due to a lack of proof that they actually work. Conversely, other doctors may in fact suggest some of these treatments, or at the very least not discourage them.

Traditional versus Integrative Medicine

Integrative medicine combines traditional medicine with other nontraditional complementary and alternative medicine (often abbreviated as CAM) with the aim of gaining benefits from both forms in order to optimize the care of a patient. CAM includes an array of treatments and products that are not part of standard, or "Western," medicine.

 Alert

Other names associated with standard medicine are mainstream, orthodox, regular, or allopathic.

Standard medical therapy is the type of medicine that is practiced by various types of medical professionals and is rooted in science. On the other hand, CAM therapy is a type of therapy that has been around for much longer than standard Western therapy. It has roots in ancient Eastern cultures and their practices and has been passed down through generations. Generally, these therapies have not been tested by the scientific community and nowadays rely more on word of mouth by individuals who have had good experiences with them. In countries such as the United States, where traditional medicine is standard, the use of CAM is nevertheless widespread and likely increasing in popularity. For example, CAM treatments have found a large following in cancer patients. Because of its promise in dealing with many types of diseases, many Lyme disease patients with continuing symptoms after their antibiotic treatment have increasingly turned to CAM. Despite a certain amount of healthy skepticism from the scientific community, some of these treatments have been shown to help a number of patients and shouldn't be immediately discounted.

Immune-Boosting Diet

Nutrition is an important aspect of good health. It is a well-known fact that if you eat well and avoid certain foods, your body will not only feel better but you will help your immune system as well. Incorporating additional foods into your diet, especially those with essential vitamins and minerals, can also result in added benefits to your body. Many people with long-term Lyme disease symptoms have switched to a more nutritious diet to help improve their symptoms, in particular inflammation.

Pro- and Anti-Inflammatory Foods

Certain foods lead to more inflammation in your body, especially in your stomach. Because inflammation causes symptoms of Lyme disease, many people say that an anti-inflammatory diet can help people with the disease. Some of the major foods or food products that people are advised to omit from their diet are:

- **Refined sugars:** These are found in various sweets, such as candy, cookies, and pastries, as well as cereals, sodas and fruit drinks, processed foods, condiments, salad dressing, barbecue sauce, pasta sauces, and canned fruit and vegetables. Basically anything that adds sugar into the recipe is going to have refined sugars.
- **Gluten:** This is a general name for proteins naturally found in wheat, rye, and barley. Gluten is found in many foods and has been implicated as a cause of a wide array of gastrointestinal diseases, such as celiac disease and leaky gut syndrome.
- **Dairy products:** These include any milk-based products, such as cheese, yogurt, or butter. Dairy products can cause gastrointestinal problems including stomach pain, constipation, and diarrhea.
- **Cooking oils:** Many of these contain polyunsaturated fatty acids, which, along with increasing inflammation, can increase the likelihood of heart disease and cancer.
- **Trans fats:** These are found in fried foods and foods prepared with partially hydrogenated oil, margarine, and vegetable shortening.

Conversely, many foods are recommended for their supposed anti-inflammatory components and may be beneficial. Some of these include:

- **Omega-3 fatty acids:** These are found in oily fish, such as salmon or tuna, and help prevent a wide variety of diseases.
- **Leafy green vegetables:** These include collard greens, spinach, and kale. They contain antioxidants, vitamin C,

carotenoids, and flavonoids that can help protect against cellular damage.

- **Coconut water:** This is believed to have antioxidant properties.
- **Fermented vegetables:** This includes foods such as raw sauerkraut or pickles. They're believed to improve the gut microbiome and help in digestion.
- **Various fruits:** Fruits said to help with inflammation include pineapples, apples, lemons, and tart cherries.
- **Extra-virgin olive oil:** This has many different compounds that possibly have antimicrobial properties to help reduce inflammation.
- **Garlic:** This also is believed to have some antimicrobial properties.
- **Lean meats:** These have antioxidant compounds that prevent cell damage.

The efficacy of many of these foods in improving your health and boosting your immune system has been well described in various scientific studies. Some other foods that have been touted more through positive experiences haven't been studied as much, so their benefits may not be as clear. Nevertheless, the Internet contains a vast amount of information about how some of these foods can be used to maintain a healthier lifestyle.

Supplements and Biotics

There are a number of supplements you can take that may have a positive effect on your body, including multivitamins, essential fatty acids derived from plant and fish oils, ubiquinone (otherwise known as CoQ10), vitamin B, magnesium, and aloe vera super juice. Probiotics and prebiotics are also very useful for helping with your health. Probiotics are live microorganisms that, when ingested in the right amounts, provide some health benefits. These "good" microbes most commonly include lactic acid bacteria and bifido-bacteria. They adjust the microbial balance of the gastrointestinal tract, and can have anti-inflammatory effects within the intestines. Prebiotics consist of some nondigestible food ingredients, mainly certain sugars, that are a source of nutrients for the probiotics. They stimulate the growth and activity of the "good" bacteria in the digestive tract and help grant benefits to your health.

Homeopathy

Many people think that homeopathy and herbal medicine are the same. They aren't. Homeopathy, also known as homeopathic medicine, is based on the idea that the body can heal itself. Central to homeopathy is the idea that "like cures like." Pills or liquid mixtures that contain a tiny trace of some active ingredient used to treat a disease are essential in homeopathy, with the active ingredient being something that has a direct role in causing the disease you're trying to cure. Only just enough of the ingredient is provided because this treatment is primarily aimed at starting the healing process, which your own body then finishes.

Homeopathic preparations include substances obtained from many different sources, including animals, plants, and minerals. In addition, some homeopathic preparations are called "nosodes," which are prepared from a sample containing a pathogen. The sample is first sterilized and then diluted many times over, to the point where very little of the actual specimen is left. For example, the active ingredient in a homeopathic treatment for Lyme disease may be a minute amount of *B. burgdorferi* itself pulled from a blood sample of a patient with Lyme.

There are two main categories of homeopathic treatment: treatments for acute, or recent, infection, and treatments for chronic infection. The use of homeopathy has been explored by Lyme disease patients for the treatment of both stages. Lyme disease homeopathic treatment includes nosodes that contain *B. burgdorferi* and sometimes other tick-borne agents. Homeopathic remedies are selected based on the patient's symptoms. Many people with Lyme disease use homeopathic care alongside other CAM approaches and standard medical therapy.

Acupuncture

Acupuncture therapy is a very old remedy. It originated in China, with some descriptions of it dating back to 300 B.C., although it likely began even earlier. Acupuncture therapy consists of a trained professional inserting approximately five to twenty small needles into specific sites of the body. The small size of the needles results in minimal to no pain when they are inserted. The patient and the needles are then left to wait for ten to twenty minutes, after which the needles are removed.

The historical concept of acupuncture is based on the concept of meridians, or qi (pronounced "chee"). The qi is believed to be a vital life force energy that circulates through the body and needs to be balanced. An imbalance of qi will cause blood flow stagnation and may result in various diseases or injuries. Despite its long-standing acceptance in many Eastern cultures, traditional Western medicine has found no evidence for the existence of these meridians.

People receive acupuncture treatments to deal with a wide array of health problems, many that include various types of pain. There are no explanations for how acupuncture works, at least not in terms of Western medical treatment. One possibility is that it causes your body to release endorphins, your body's natural chemicals that produce an overall better feeling and may reduce pain. Because of its association with pain relief, many individuals have explored the use of acupuncture in treating the symptoms associated with Lyme disease. It has been used to treat joint pain, arthritis, and nerve damage, and some patients have reported very satisfactory results following acupuncture treatment. Some people have also used a technique called cupping, along with acupuncture, for pain relief. Cupping involves placing suction cups of various shapes and sizes on a person's skin in order to increase blood flow.

❓ Question

What is a placebo and the "placebo effect"?
A placebo is something that may appear to be a real medical treatment but really isn't. Placebos don't have any active ingredients that improve your health and are used by researchers to help them understand how the effects of a real drug compare to the effects on people who only think they are getting the drug. Sometimes people can get better while taking the placebo, which is known as the "placebo effect." Because their mind thinks they should be getting better thanks to the "drug," their body begins the healing process.

Acupuncture treatment has gained a substantial acceptance in the United States and many people are aware of the existence of this therapy. However, there has been no clear scientific evidence that acupuncture is, in fact, effective. As with most of the alternative treatments described in this chapter, there are not many studies comparing the effect of the acupuncture therapy in patients with pain against similar patients who did not receive the treatment. For some conditions, such as asthma and allergies, acupuncture treatment may not be any more effective that a placebo. However, the treatment is generally very safe with limited side effects, especially if performed by a certified acupuncturist. Thus, any pain relief that comes with acupuncture treatment is simply a much needed, welcome effect with very little risk.

Helpful Herbs

Most herbal medicines originate from China and India, as well as some ancient European cultures. Although primarily associated with plants, these occasionally also include certain animal products. Herbal medications can be eaten or drunk, applied directly onto the skin in oil form, or inhaled through aromatherapy. There is a belief that herbal therapy can provide a safe alternative treatment to the antibiotics that have severe side effects. Herbs can provide a number of antimicrobial properties and some are believed to be anti-inflammatory, which would help greatly with Lyme disease. That is not surprising, as many known antimicrobial compounds originate from plants and plant products. The use of multiple herbs can be synergistic, meaning that using them together will be more effective than using an individual herb alone. Some people advocate herbal therapy for the reduction of Lyme disease symptoms. These treatments are usually prepared as mixtures in order to provide the maximum benefit to the patient. Depending on the mixture, herbal medicine is said to have antimicrobial effects, help in detoxification and boosting the immune system, provide necessary nutrients, and improve heart function.

Meditation and Yoga

Some individuals turn to meditation and yoga as a way of coping with the symptoms of Lyme disease. Yoga is an ancient Indian workout of both the mind and body that goes back thousands of years. It combines strengthening and stretching poses to create a physical, mental, and spiritual workout that is believed to relieve the stiffness, pain, and inflammation associated with Lyme disease. Breathing and meditation have also been suggested to alleviate both the physical and mental pain. Through yoga, patients with PTLDS can be more in tune with their body. It can help them relax, lower their anxiety and insomnia, or energize them to fight against depression and fatigue. Regular yoga sessions may also help in keeping any persistent pain at a manageable level.

The Effects on Lyme Disease

So, do any of these therapies really work? The answer is sometimes; it may depend on your belief system. For the majority of these treatments, there is no scientific evidence that they reduce the symptoms associated with Lyme disease. In fact, some may even be the direct opposite of what standard medicine would tell you is a useful treatment. The Internet contains a number of success stories associated with some of these treatments. However, most of these are individual descriptions, and there is no evidence that any of these treatments performs any better than a placebo. But if you believe that using these treatments will help you, regardless of what standard medicine says, then trying them may be beneficial in the long run.

Treatments to Avoid

Patients suffering from symptoms after their treatment has ended are often at a crossroads. They have exhausted their medical options and yet they still don't feel better. Because medicine can't really help at this point, the lack of any recommended options for treatment can be very disheartening. This can lead some people to begin exploring alternative, unorthodox treatments. There are any number of different therapies that your typical doctor would not recommend, yet people still regularly try them. What are these treatments, and how do they work?

Like almost everything in this day and age, the Internet can provide an answer. A quick Internet search using certain phrases, such as "alternative Lyme disease therapy," will introduce you to a wide array of treatments that claim to cure chronic Lyme disease. In fact, many of the providers of these so-called treatments specifically target chronic Lyme disease patients because this is the group that is most likely to seek alternative treatments that go against the medically accepted recommendations. However, none of these alternative treatments have been shown to work and, in many cases, can be seriously dangerous.

Some of these dangerous and completely ineffective treatments include:

Treatments Using Various Forms of Energy and Radiation

- **Ultraviolet light therapy:** This procedure includes taking the patients' blood out of the body, exposing it to ultraviolet light, and then feeding it back into the body. This therapy is claimed to be able to kill the bacteria that is in your blood.
- **Low-level laser therapy, or "cold" therapy:** This treatment applies low-level lasers to different body parts and claims to relieve pain.
- **Photon therapy:** This treatment uses machines that emit light into your skin, which supposedly forces bacteria out of your cells, where they can then be destroyed by the immune system. Some claim that this therapy has a 96 percent cure rate for Lyme disease.
- **Pulsed electromagnetic field, or PEMF therapy:** This therapy consists of a machine that sends sound-wave vibrations to your body.
- **Rife machine therapy:** The Rife machine delivers electromagnetic energy to the body and is claimed to stimulate it to make it healthier and provide a more capable environment for killing pathogens.
- **Magnetic therapy:** This therapy claims that applying magnets to various parts of the body produces a healthier environment at these body parts that can more easily kill diseases. One such therapy recommends that you sleep and rest on a bed of seventy magnets.

Oxygen Therapies

- **Hyperbaric oxygen chamber therapy:** This treatment consists of placing a patient in a hyperbaric oxygen chamber, where the oxygen pressure is greater than the oxygen pressure outside. It is claimed that this treatment has beneficial effects on the immune system, which can then better fight *B. burgdorferi* infections.
- **Ozone therapy:** This therapy consists of introduction of the compound ozone into the body. Ozone occurs naturally in the atmosphere, and it's claimed that therapy with ozone can improve the function of the immune system and relieve the persistent symptoms of chronic Lyme disease. The treatment is performed by mixing ozone with other gases or liquids and then introducing it into the body in various uncomfortable ways.

Treatment with Metals

- **Mercury detoxification:** This therapy claims that mercury toxicity often accompanies chronic Lyme disease. According to the theory, in order to see improvement in Lyme disease symptoms, you need to remove mercury from your system. Treatments include metal chelation therapy, in which various compounds are used to bind mercury and eliminate it from the bloodstream.
- **Silver:** Therapy with silver is said to help the immune system destroy the bacteria. It is usually available in a "colloidal" form, which consists of silver particles resuspended in a liquid solution. Silver nanoparticles, which are even smaller particles, are also now being recommended.

- **Bismuth:** Bismuth is claimed to have antimicrobial properties, including the ability to kill cystic forms of *B. burgdorferi*.

Various Biological Therapies

- **Urotherapy:** This therapy suggests that drinking your own urine can improve your health.
- **Enemas:** This therapy claims that enemas, largely used for detoxification, will help the immune system.
- **Bee venom:** Some claim this has antimicrobial and anti-inflammatory properties.
- **Many different steroids:** These are promoted as helping with adrenal fatigue, an unproven claim that the adrenal glands can get exhausted and cannot produce enough hormones.
- **Apheresis:** Similar to ultraviolet light treatment, only without the light, this technique involves taking blood out, filtering it, and reinfusing it into the body. It has been promoted to remove toxins.
- **Miracle mineral solution:** This solution is essentially made up of 28 percent bleach and water and has been promoted as a cure for a wide array of diseases.
- **Stem cell transplant:** This is promoted to repair cellular damage caused by Lyme disease.
- **Other medicines:** Drugs clinically not used for Lyme disease treatment include olmesartan, dimethyl sulfoxide, naltrexone, or lithium orotate salt.

The main warning about these treatments is the fact that none of them have been properly, scientifically evaluated. For a treatment to be approved by the FDA, it is must pass rigorous testing for both safety and effectiveness. There is no such review for these alternative treatments. So why do people try them? Some people with severe, debilitating symptoms just want to get better and are willing to try anything. They hope that the treatment, no matter how unorthodox, will somehow work and take away their pain. Others may be seduced by marketing strategies that claim fantastic results, including high cure rates. Then there are others who may simply distrust doctors and scientists and feel compelled to try alternative means of therapy. It's true that some patients improve after these treatments and believe that they were effective. Whether the treatment itself is the reason for the improvement is debatable; the improvements may simply be from the placebo effect.

ⓔ Alert

The phrase "natural" is often applied to many alternative treatments to differentiate them from "chemical" treatments. However, this is often intentionally misleading, as everything is made up of chemicals. Conversely, many things that are toxic to you can be natural. For example, most of the deadliest poisons in the world are natural. Even though something may be "natural," that does not mean it will automatically be good for you.

Even if you have no other options for getting better, you still risk a lot if you choose to use these alternative treatments. For starters, many of these treatments are incredibly expensive, with some of the machines listed earlier costing several thousands of dollars. More important, many of these treatments are highly dangerous and potentially even lethal. Some of them are so dangerous that not only does the FDA not endorse them, they have explicit warnings against their use for Lyme disease.

If you are one of the PTLDS patients who is at a crossroads and don't know what to do next, it is understandable that you may be tempted to try any one of these unorthodox treatments. If you are, make sure that you do your homework first. So how do you look out for potential scams? Be wary of any alternative treatment that advertises amazing cure rates and uses big, scientific-sounding words to back up its claims. Try to find real evidence that the treatment works, not just word of mouth. Find out if any descriptions of this treatment have been published in a scientific journal. Has there been real clinical testing of the treatment? And find out if the treatment is licensed, and if so, what has it been licensed for? Some treatments may be licensed, but not for treatment of infectious diseases such as Lyme disease. At the end of the day, having all the necessary information will help you make the best decision about your treatment.

Summary

Antibiotics are the standard treatment for all stages of Lyme disease. The most frequently prescribed antibiotics for Lyme disease are doxycycline, amoxicillin, and cefuroxime axetil, which are all taken in pill form. The length of the treatment can range between ten days and three weeks, and will ultimately depend on your doctor. For late Lyme disease, patients are often given a second dosage. Patients with severe symptoms receive an IV antibiotic called ceftriaxone.

The treatment is very effective for most patients and resistance to these drugs has not been seen. However, sometimes the treatment doesn't work and some patients continue to have a subjective illness long after treatment, such as PTLDS or chronic Lyme disease. Based on the belief that the bacteria are often not fully eradicated after antibiotics, some in the Lyme disease community have advocated for a longer antibiotic treatment. To investigate this, four major studies have looked at the benefits of prolonged antibiotic treatment in patients with persistent symptoms. In two of the studies, the long-term treatment was not any better than the currently recommended one. In the other two, some benefits were seen, but the risk associated with the continued treatment outweighed the benefits. As a result, the official guidelines for treating Lyme disease discourage prolonged antibiotic treatment. Some members of the community disagree with both the guidelines and with the results of the four studies they were based on, believing that the studies were flawed. Some doctors advocate prolonged treatment for patients when the symptoms do not go away.

In part because of the controversies and the lack of adequate treatment, patients with PTLDS or chronic Lyme disease have sought out alternative treatments to lessen their symptoms. These include herbal medicine, homeopathy, acupuncture, and dietary alternatives. Although the actual benefits of these treatments are not known, some patients claim to get better. However, in addition to these treatments, there are a number of treatments that are much more unconventional and potentially dangerous that patients need to be aware of.

CHAPTER 7

Lyme Disease Advocacy

Lyme disease has some of the strongest advocacy groups found in this country. A quick online search will reveal a wide array of groups whose missions promote awareness of the disease, raise funds for research, and lobby for patients' rights. Many patients, particularly ones who have been diagnosed with chronic Lyme disease, have joined these groups and have made substantial impacts, both locally in their communities and nationally through influencing legislature. The number of these advocacy groups appears to be increasing. However, these groups tend to also include some of the most vocal proponents of the existence of chronic Lyme disease. As a result, many of these groups are at odds with members of the scientific community by promoting their alternative view of Lyme disease.

The Lyme Community

The most recent estimates coming out of the CDC place the number of Lyme disease cases at roughly 300,000 each year. This was a staggering increase of a disease that until recently was reported at just one tenth that amount. It was also validation in the eyes of many Lyme disease activists who were convinced that this illness was much more widespread than most people thought. For years, many of these individuals have felt that scientists and many physicians marginalized the magnitude of the disease and the suffering associated with it. Particularly, they felt that many of the decisions that were made regarding diagnosis and treatment came without their input, by individuals who were not aware of the extent of the overall problem.

Initially, local support groups for Lyme disease patients were started in the 1980s to educate patients and physicians, provide support for patients, and raise funds to help fight the illness. Many of these groups were soon succeeded by more national organizations, a number of which are proponents of the existence of chronic Lyme disease. They generally consist of patients and their families, their doctors, and a small number of scientists, and they tend to have a strong Internet presence. Many individuals have blogs where they share their opinions and the newest scientific findings surrounding Lyme disease, and quite a few of the groups hold scientific meetings of their own. They have received celebrity endorsements and formed political lobbies. As a result, these groups have made a large impact in bringing the concept of chronic Lyme disease to the mainstream.

Lyme Disease Advocacy Causes

Many individuals who become Lyme disease activists do so because of their own past or current experience with the disease. Others are parents who have seen their children bedridden for months or years. Some advocates include physicians who, upon getting the disease or seeing how it affects others, have changed their views on how it should be treated.

The primary aims of various Lyme disease organizations are to help prevent Lyme disease, improve the diagnosis of the disease, and make it easier to cure for everyone. This involves better education and research into the disease. For chronic Lyme disease advocacy groups, it also involves the acceptance of this condition by the mainstream public.

Change in Guidelines for Lyme Disease Treatment

Most Lyme disease advocacy groups want significantly more say over how the disease is treated than they currently have. This includes forcing changes to the existing IDSA guidelines for treatment of Lyme disease as well as any resulting persistent symptoms. Many members of Lyme disease advocacy groups believe that the current guidelines are not well supported by scientific evidence, are not appropriate for all Lyme disease patients, and should be revised to be more inclusive of patients with chronic Lyme disease. Because there is no other treatment available for persistent symptoms, advocates believe that patients should have the right to choose any treatment they want, even if it includes long-term antibiotic therapy. A major sticking point is the fact that insurance companies use the current IDSA guidelines to make their decisions regarding whether or not they will cover the cost of any Lyme disease treatments. A substantial part of chronic Lyme disease treatment, in particular long-term antibiotic therapy, is seen by insurance companies as unproven. As a result, many insurance companies decline to cover the costs associated with it, which can have profound effects on patients' finances.

In order to bring more light to this cause, advocacy groups have organized rallies in cities all over the United States, some in front of the White House. Other rallies have been held outside of buildings where the IDSA was meeting in order to protest their guidelines for treatment. Some rallies have included "die-ins," where groups pretend to be dead to show the seriousness of the disease to people walking past.

Advocacy for Lyme-Literate Doctors

A common feeling for many people within the Lyme advocacy community is that most doctors do not understand their condition.

Some feel that they have been let down by the medical profession, particularly in instances where the doctors appear to not fully believe the symptoms the patients are describing. They are put off by what they perceive as minimization of their pain and suffering and object to the idea that nothing can be done if antibiotics don't work. Many patients wind up going to multiple doctors and still feel dissatisfied with their care.

These experiences have led to the strong movement toward supporting Lyme-literate doctors. These doctors frequently do not go along with the established dogma for treating Lyme disease and claim that they can properly diagnose and treat patients with chronic Lyme disease. Many of these doctors promote a treatment using multiple rounds of antibiotics. Because such treatment is often seen as unnecessary and dangerous by the medical community at large, especially in cases where patients have no evidence of actually having Lyme disease, a number of Lyme-literate doctors have lost their medical license for practicing medicine outside of the established guidelines. In response, many advocates have taken up the cause of protecting these doctors. Due to actions of advocacy groups, several states have passed laws that protect doctors from disciplinary action in their treatment of Lyme disease, and similar bills have been introduced in other states. For patients who are looking for such a doctor, some Lyme disease advocacy websites will provide referrals to Lyme-literate doctors.

Fund-Raising

As with most nonprofit organizations, Lyme disease groups employ a variety of fund-raising methods. Many ask that you make a monetary donation. Alternatively, you can become a member of any number of groups, which carries a price but can also include various gifts and access to more information. In addition, various Lyme disease advocacy groups organize fund-raising events that are held throughout the country. These include sporting events, such as Lyme golfing tournaments, various Lyme runs or walks, and endurance events such as marathons. There are many fundraising social events such as wine tastings, art shows, benefit dinners, and concerts. The proceeds of these events are being used to fund a wide variety of education, patient care, and research programs.

Many of the funds raised go directly to help people suffering from Lyme disease. Because of the high cost of healthcare associated with it, particularly for uninsured patients, various advocacy groups have created programs that help parents without insurance cover the cost of their children's Lyme disease treatment. Some groups also offer financial assistance for Lyme diagnostic testing.

Lyme disease advocacy groups also use these funds to help with research, which is often one of their main causes. This includes lobbying the federal government to increase the amount of funding toward tick-borne disease research, which is very inadequate right now. Some of the national Lyme disease support organizations have also raised and distributed millions of dollars in research grants, with several individual grants giving more than one hundred thousand dollars per year. Many of the grants go to established researchers while others are available for new scientists with unique research ideas. Some groups offer these grants each year. These funds have been used to pay for postdoctoral fellowships, research assistants, and expensive state-of-the-art equipment. They have been used to create a Lyme disease "biobank"—a large group of blood samples from patients with Lyme disease that are made available to other researchers for their studies—and to cofound a research center for Lyme and tick-borne diseases at Columbia University. Several groups also organize scientific meetings where original research is presented and discussed.

Lyme Disease Education

Many Lyme disease organizations provide free brochures on a wide variety of subjects around Lyme disease such as tick awareness or general facts about Lyme disease. Many groups maintain a strong presence in various communities through outreach programs and various Lyme disease awareness initiatives. They provide or participate in public forums that present information about Lyme disease. Some maintain a toll-free information line with facts about the disease. Several groups have developed education platforms that can be used in school, such as presentations and prevention videos that can be found on their websites and interactive curricula for different age groups. These include various activities that can be added into existing basic science or health curricula for school districts. Some groups also provide educational programs for doctors to learn more about how to diagnose and treat Lyme disease and other tick-borne diseases.

Support Groups

A number of Lyme disease organizations provide information on how to join support groups. These are not limited to the United States; many of these groups exist in other countries as well. These support groups can range from online forums to local community-level programs. Many patients with PTLDS or chronic Lyme disease describe how receiving support from others who are suffering through a similar condition can have a positive effect on their morale. Some finally feel that their symptoms are real, and it can help them cope and stop feeling isolated. Some patients also feel satisfaction from being able to share their experience and perhaps help educate others who have just been diagnosed with the illness.

Online Resources

If you've had Lyme disease and are looking to join a support group to discuss your experiences, you can search the Internet and you will find a number of links to Lyme disease support groups in every state. Likewise, if you are looking to make a donation, many organizations encourage members to donate. You can find some of the most well-known Lyme disease groups in Appendix A: Further Resources.

Online Misinformation

Unfortunately, as is true with much of the information found on the Internet, many of the websites and blogs within the Lyme disease community contain a great deal of misinformation. You have to be wary of much of the information that you read regarding this disease online. Regardless of whether you believe in chronic Lyme disease or not, propagating misinformation and providing unproven claims as scientific fact only promotes even more misunderstanding of this disease. Make sure that the websites you use to help you in your fight against Lyme disease, whether for education or advocacy, are reputable and reliable.

✅ Fact

An example of obvious misinformation that you can find on the web are claims that *B. burgdorferi* was made by humans or that it came from Plum Island, an island off the coast of Long Island. This is biologically impossible and false.

Scientific Concerns with Lyme Disease Advocacy

Many members within the scientific community view several aspects of Lyme disease advocacy with apprehension and as part of an overall anti-science movement. The original concept of Lyme disease support groups was to serve as a source of information for the patients and the public. However, some scientists believe that they have evolved into organizations that promote the concept of chronic Lyme disease based on unproven theories and endorse clinical services that have no basis in scientific fact. This has led to some Lyme disease activists organizing their own scientific conferences, publishing their own scientific journal, and funding research by Lyme-literate physicians. This is an unfortunate development because it has resulted in the creation of two distinct groups that fundamentally differ on their views of several aspects of Lyme disease.

The battle between the Lyme disease advocates and the scientific community started in the early 1990s. At that time, Lyme disease advocacy groups, along with some Lyme-literate doctors, began accusing university scientists and public health officials of intentionally underreporting and underdiagnosing Lyme disease. Disputes with health insurance companies, which would deny payment for long-term treatments, were often blamed on academic physicians. Many of these doctors were accused of conflicts of interest. The controversies even reached the political arena, with the US Congress holding hearings about Lyme disease. Several congressmen investigated Lyme disease research programs within the Centers for Disease Control and Prevention (CDC) and the National Institutes of Health (NIH). The attorney general of Connecticut, a long-time supporter of Lyme disease activism, even threatened the IDSA with an antitrust lawsuit, though no lawsuit was filed. And probably the most well-known occurrence of Lyme disease activism having a major impact on the scientific aspect of the disease was the failure of the Lyme disease vaccine in the early 2000s.

LYMErix

The best way to prevent Lyme disease is to prevent tick bites. Another method could be through vaccination, which is a common way of preventing diseases. Unfortunately, there are no Lyme disease vaccines out on the market today. However, there was one available in the 1990s called LYMErix before it was pulled just three years after being released.

In the early to mid-1990s, two pharmaceutical companies, alongside some of the leading Lyme disease scientists and clinicians in the country, developed two similar Lyme disease vaccines. Both vaccines were based on a *B. burgdorferi* protein called OspA, and both were tested in clinical trials to see if they were effective and worth putting on the market. Only one of the vaccines, LYMErix, was submitted for FDA approval and it was introduced into the market in 1999. Upon its initial release, there was a lot of positive media coverage and LYMErix was thought to be highly beneficial.

⊛ Essential

Vaccines work by tricking your immune system into reacting as if you are infected with the actual pathogen. After getting the vaccine, your body will make antibodies to the vaccine and eliminate it while also ensuring that it will "remember" the pathogen. Sometime later in the future, when you do get infected with the actual pathogen, your immune system will have the antibodies ready to eliminate the infection immediately.

However, there were several limitations of LYMErix. It was only about 80 percent effective, meaning that about 20 percent of vaccinated people could still get Lyme disease. To get the full protection, you needed to receive three doses of the vaccine: an initial dose, a dose one month later, and then another twelve months after that. There was also a possibility that on top of these three doses, you may have needed additional booster shots, perhaps as often as every single year. The vaccine was also never tested in children, which meant they couldn't have been vaccinated. Finally, there was evidence that a portion of OspA was similar to a protein found in humans. As a result, there was a fear that the vaccine could potentially trigger an autoimmune response and your immune system would attack the body even without an infection from *B. burgdorferi.*

Within a year of being on the market, there were reports of side effects of the vaccination. Some people who were vaccinated complained of various problems, mostly arthritis, which they believed to have been caused by the vaccine. This began a quick change in public opinion against the vaccine. A number of Lyme disease advocacy groups, who initially were supportive of the vaccine, began a campaign against it, because of major concerns over its safety. Some claimed that the vaccine itself could result in a Lyme disease–like illness.

 Fact

Dogs can frequently be infected with *B. burgdorferi,* although most do not become ill. Although the human Lyme disease vaccine is not on the market, vaccines for dogs are available, and dog owners in common Lyme disease areas have the option to vaccinate their pets.

A year after entering the market, the vaccine manufacturer was sued by a law firm representing 121 people who claimed they had significant side effects from the vaccine. The FDA performed an extensive examination of all the data regarding the vaccine, but found that there did not appear to be any unusual side effects. For example, the rate of people who complained of arthritis after vaccination was the same as in the general population. However, during hearings regarding the safety of the vaccine, a number of advocates spoke strongly against it. All of these developments resulted in a large amount of predominantly negative media coverage. As a result, sales of the vaccine dropped dramatically in 2001. In early 2002, the vaccine's manufacturer took it off the market, citing poor sales. Because of this, many scientists were convinced that activism against the vaccine was a major reason for its failure.

Summary

The Lyme disease community includes several groups that have been founded with a goal of promoting awareness of Lyme disease and helping patients deal with this illness. These groups have had a large impact on educating the public about the dangers of ticks and the diseases they carry. They have raised millions of dollars to support a wide variety of research projects and to help with health-care costs. By forming support groups, they have also been essential in helping patients deal with their suffering.

Many of these groups have also taken a strong stand in opposition to the current methods for diagnosis and treatment of Lyme disease. This has led to the formation of two distinct factions associated with Lyme disease. One consists of medical experts who set the guidelines for diagnosis and treatment, and the other is mostly advocacy groups that disagree with many of these methods and actively campaign to change them. These advocacy groups have been successful in helping pass laws that protect chronic Lyme disease treatment, and their strong opposition to the Lyme disease vaccine resulted in its quick withdrawal. As a result, some scientists have been concerned that the views of some of the advocacy groups can have a negative impact on science.

CHAPTER 8

Potential Coinfections

Imagine finding an engorged blacklegged nymph somewhere on your body. After removing the tick, and having read this book, you're worried that you may have just gotten Lyme disease. You know that it may take at least a few days before you start developing any signs and symptoms. The wait can be nerve wracking, so you decide that you can't wait, and you send the tick away for testing. In a day or so, you get the results: the tick was not infected with *B. burgdorferi*. You breathe a sigh of relief and move on. Then, a few days later, you begin to feel ill. You go to a doctor and tell her that you were bitten by a tick but that you tested it for *B. burgdorferi* and it was negative. There is no way you can have Lyme disease, can you? The doctor suggests taking a blood sample and sending it away for testing anyway. A day later the test results are in and the doctor calls you to let you know that you do, in fact, have a tick-borne disease. You're confused; how can you have a tick-borne disease if the tick that bit you was not infected with *B. burgdorferi*?

Coinfections

Lyme disease is usually the biggest concern of people who reside in areas common to ticks. Considering how common Lyme disease can be, that is completely reasonable. Unfortunately, even if you get bitten by a tick that does not have *B. burgdorferi*, there is always a possibility that you were exposed to one of the many other pathogens that ticks can transmit. Right now, there are about twenty or so tick-transmitted pathogens that have been linked to human disease throughout the United States and the list keeps growing. It seems every year or so, a new tick-borne pathogen is discovered. Some of these pathogens are transmitted by tick species other than the blacklegged tick, such as lone star ticks or American dog ticks. And then there are the blacklegged ticks themselves.

Being responsible for transmission of Lyme disease makes the blacklegged ticks a big enough problem. Unfortunately, Lyme disease is not the only disease that blacklegged ticks are associated with. They are known to carry and transmit at least five different human pathogens, which is the most out of any of tick species found in the United States. You already know about Lyme disease. The other four are babesiosis, anaplasmosis, Powassan virus disease, and *Borrelia miyamotoi* disease. Babesiosis and anaplasmosis are not uncommon, with each disease occurring in more than a thousand people every year. Although Powassan virus disease and *Borrelia miyamotoi* disease are still pretty rare, they unfortunately appear to be rising in frequency, along with anaplasmosis and babesiosis. If you happen to find an engorged blacklegged tick somewhere on your body, Lyme disease is not the only thing you need to worry about.

Babesiosis

Babesiosis is a disease that occurs worldwide and is caused by an infection by an organism called *Babesia*. In addition to human disease, babesiosis is also a significant problem for livestock, in particularly cattle. To separate human and animal disease, human infections are often referred to as human babesiosis. In the United States, human disease is primarily caused by a species of *Babesia* called *Babesia microti*. Two other species, *Babesia duncani* on the Pacific Coast and *Babesia divergens* in the mid-South, can also infect people but are very rare, and the vast majority of human infections in the United States are believed to be by *B. microti*.

Unlike many of the tick-borne diseases discussed in this book, babesiosis has a well-described history. *Babesia* was first discovered in 1888 as the cause of a disease in cattle called Texas cattle fever. Soon after, in 1893, Texas cattle fever was revealed to be transmitted by ticks. This was the very first time any infectious disease was shown to be transmitted by any arthropod.

 Fact

Babesiosis is extremely important to the cattle industry. If cattle become infected with Texas cattle fever, they generally die three out of every four times. For that reason, the ticks responsible, called cattle ticks, were eradicated in the United States in the first half of the twentieth century.

In the past, human babesiosis was not as big a concern in the United States as it has been within the past decade. In fact, human babesiosis was not even a reportable disease until 2011, meaning cases were generally not even reported. In the 1970s and early 1980s, babesiosis was confined to a few areas in the Northeast, particularly Long Island, New York, and several New England islands such as Martha's Vineyard and Nantucket Island. Since then, babesiosis has expanded north, south, and west, very similarly to how Lyme disease expanded from the mid-1970s onward. In comparison to Lyme disease, however, the expansion has been much slower, and babesiosis is still very rarely reported in areas away from the Atlantic Coast.

Alert

Babesiosis is not a rare disease, particularly in tick-endemic areas. In 2011, the first year babesiosis was a reportable disease, 1,126 cases were reported. By 2014, this number had increased to 1,744.

Nearly 95 percent of babesiosis cases occur in seven states. Five are in the Northeast—New York, New Jersey, Massachusetts,

Connecticut, and Rhode Island—while the other two, Minnesota and Wisconsin, are located in the north-central part of the country. Other cases are occasionally reported along the northeastern Atlantic Coast from Maine down to Maryland, and some sporadic cases caused by other *Babesia* species occur in northern California, Washington, Missouri, and Kentucky.

✅ Fact

Babesia organisms look very similar to the pathogens that cause malaria. When looking at blood samples under the microscope, the two organisms look almost identical, both appearing as rings inside red blood cells. Only trained scientists can tell them apart.

B. microti is transmitted by the bites of blacklegged ticks. As with Lyme disease, the ticks typically get infected as larvae when they feed on an infected white-footed mouse, which is also the main reservoir for *B. microti*. Infection rates of ticks can vary depending on the area. In areas with a long history of babesiosis, they can be high, with up to one out of every five nymphal ticks being infected. In other areas, typically further away from the Atlantic Coast, as few as 1 percent of the ticks can be infected. As is the case with Lyme disease, infection with *B. microti* does not occur quickly; it takes about thirty-six to seventy-two hours for an attached tick to transmit *B. microti* to a new host. Although reported year-round, the majority of cases of babesiosis are reported in June through August, with a peak in July, due to the bites of infected nymphal ticks.

Transfusions and Babesiosis

In addition to being transmitted by ticks, you can also get babesiosis through blood transfusions. Blood donors are currently not tested for infection with *Babesia* due to lack of an adequate test, and occasionally people who have the disease but no symptoms will donate blood, which is then transfused to other patients. *B. microti* is the most frequent microbial pathogen transmitted through blood transfusions in the United States, with more than 170 reported cases. Because the blacklegged tick is not needed for this, babesiosis caused by transfusions can occur throughout the year and in all areas of the United States. Because many people who receive blood transfusions often have weak immune systems, about one fifth of babesiosis cases that have occurred through blood transfusion have resulted in the patient dying. Babesiosis can also be transmitted from a mother to her unborn baby if she has the disease while pregnant.

Essential

Babesia are not bacteria; they are unicellular eukaryotic parasites, meaning they consist of one cell that is somewhat similar to our cells. As a result, many antibiotics that target bacteria do not affect *Babesia*.

Signs and Symptoms of Babesiosis

Babesiosis is a blood disease. After transmission from the tick, this pathogen infects and kills red blood cells. The symptoms of babesiosis are the result of the damage from the destroyed cells as well as the inflammatory response of the immune system. Infection with *B. microti* often does not result in any symptoms, particularly in young, healthy people. For example, about half of infected children may not show symptoms. The likelihood of the disease symptoms appearing increases with age, with the largest number of severe cases typically occurring in people between the ages of sixty and sixty-nine.

If you do have symptoms of babesiosis, they will appear around one to four weeks after the initial tick bite. They typically consist of fever, fatigue, chills, sweats, headache, body aches, loss of appetite, nausea, and joint pain. The symptoms are typically very nonspecific, and can be mistaken for a large number of other infections, including Lyme disease. Some people also have additional symptoms that include abdominal pain, vomiting, sensitivity to light, and weight loss. About half of the patients with babesiosis have severe symptoms that require hospital admission. There are several risk factors that make it more likely you will develop a severe case of babesiosis, including:

- Being over fifty years of age
- Having a weakened immune system because of other health problems, such as cancer or AIDS
- Having other health problems such as liver or kidney disease
- Missing your spleen

In patients who have these problems, babesiosis can cause many complications that potentially lead to organ failure or even death. About one-tenth of people hospitalized with babesiosis die of the disease.

Patients requiring hospitalization frequently develop additional problems from babesiosis. Because *Babesia* destroys red blood cells, it can cause anemia, which is a decrease in the number of red blood cells in the blood. Anemia occurs in more than half of babesiosis patients. The specific type associated with babesiosis is called hemolytic anemia. This can cause the skin to turn yellow, which is known as jaundice, and can also cause the patient to produce dark urine. The majority of patients also develop a condition called thrombocytopenia, which is characterized by a low platelet count. Because platelets help in blood clotting, this condition can have severe effects on the outcome of the disease due to excessive bleeding. Patients with babesiosis might also get an enlarged spleen.

Diagnosis and Treatment of Babesiosis

Babesiosis does not have unique signs and symptoms. Because of this, diagnosis of babesiosis can be difficult. If your doctor thinks you may have it, the diagnosis is usually confirmed only after sending a blood sample for analysis. The presence of the pathogen can be verified in red blood cells when a blood sample is observed under a microscope. PCR tests for *B. microti* are also available and can be used to diagnose the disease in the early stages. Serologic tests are usually only useful later on in the disease, and are mostly used to confirm a diagnosis that was made earlier in the disease with other methods. For serologic tests, generally specimens collected weeks apart are tested for an increase of antibodies to *B. microti*.

Most infected people who do not have symptoms do not require treatment. Patients with symptoms will usually receive treatment for seven to ten days with a combination of two prescription medications, either atovaquone and azithromycin together or clindamycin and quinine, which is the standard for severely ill patients. Hospitalized patients with severe cases of babesiosis may need additional therapy, including blood transfusions, mechanical ventilation, and dialysis.

Anaplasmosis

Anaplasmosis was first recognized as a human disease in 1994 under the name "human granulocytic ehrlichiosis." In 2001, the name of the pathogen that causes the disease was changed from *Ehrlichia phagocytophilum* to *Anaplasma phagocytophilum*, and the name of the disease was changed to human granulocytic anaplasmosis (abbreviated to HGA but most often called simply anaplasmosis). If you happen to come across an old article about "granulocytic ehrlichiosis," it's really the same thing as anaplasmosis. It can get a little confusing, especially because there is a different tick-borne disease called "ehrlichiosis," which is discussed in Appendix C: Infections Transmitted by Other Ticks.

Anaplasmosis occurs in North America and in Europe. In North America, the disease is caused by the bites of blacklegged ticks and can occur anywhere this tick is found. Ticks infected with *A. phagocytophilum* are not as common as ticks with *B. burgdorferi*. In some areas, in particular in the Northeast and around the Great Lakes, roughly 15 percent of nymphal blacklegged ticks and 25 percent of adult ticks are infected. In most of the other areas in the range of the blacklegged tick, less than 5 percent of nymphs are infected.

Anaplasmosis is most frequently reported in adults over forty years old. The disease is reported throughout the year, but peaks in June and July, around the time when blacklegged tick nymphs come out to feed. The majority of cases are clustered in the northeastern and north-central parts of the United States, with very few cases being reported on the West Coast. Anaplasmosis first became a nationally reportable disease in 1999, and the number of cases reported by the CDC has risen dramatically since that time. In 2000, 350 cases of anaplasmosis were reported. By 2010, this number increased to 1,761, and by 2015, it had jumped to 3,656. However, this does not include any cases where symptoms didn't appear or any undiagnosed infections, which are believed to occur frequently as well.

Signs and Symptoms of Anaplasmosis

Anaplasmosis is a blood disease, like babesiosis. However, unlike babesiosis, after it's transmitted from the tick, the bacteria infects certain types of white blood cells, not red blood cells, before killing them and producing an inflammatory reaction in your blood. Infection with *A. phagocytophilum* often doesn't show any symptoms. If you do have symptoms, they will usually begin within the first week or two after the tick bite. The symptoms typically consist of a fever, headache, muscle pain, fatigue, chills, nausea, abdominal pain, cough, and confusion. On rare occasions, some patients may also have a rash. In some people with anaplasmosis, the disease can be severe enough that they have to be admitted to the hospital. If not treated, anaplasmosis can cause life-threatening complications, including difficulty breathing, bleeding, kidney failure, and neurological problems. On rare occasions, it can also be fatal. Of the roughly 16,000 patients diagnosed with anaplasmosis since 1994, eleven have died. If you have any problems with your immune system, the disease may be more severe. In cases such as these, anaplasmosis may result in death.

✅ Fact

The name of the disease human granulocytic anaplasmosis refers to the type of cell that is affected during the disease. *A. phagocytophilum* infects a specific type of white blood cell called a granulocyte, also known as a neutrophil. Hence the name "granulocytic" anaplasmosis.

It is possible to get anaplasmosis without a tick bite. If you're pregnant and have anaplasmosis, you can pass the infection on to your fetus. In addition, at least eight cases of anaplasmosis have been reported through a transfusion with infected blood. It may also be possible to become infected with anaplasmosis by coming in contact with the blood of an infected animal or patient. People at risk for such an infection can easily prevent it by taking simple precautions such as wearing gloves.

Diagnosis of anaplasmosis may be difficult because of the lack of specific signs and symptoms that are unique to this disease. Your doctor may suspect you have anaplasmosis if you live in one of the areas where the disease is common, you remember being recently bitten by a tick, and you do not have the EM rash, which would lead to a diagnosis of Lyme disease instead. To confirm a diagnosis of anaplasmosis, the doctor will draw a sample of your blood and send it to a laboratory for analysis. However, you will be started on antibiotics immediately because it may take a day or longer for the test results to come in, and the treatment will be more effective the earlier in the disease you are. You will usually be prescribed doxycycline, and required to take it for seven to fourteen days. However, if you are pregnant, doxycycline is not given, so another antibiotic, rifampin, may be prescribed instead. If you are diagnosed and begin treatment within the first five days of the disease, the fever will generally go away within twenty-four to seventy-two hours. Even without treatment, nearly all patients recover completely within sixty days, although a small group may continue to have symptoms for weeks, even after treatment. These symptoms include a headache, weakness, and a general feeling of discomfort. However, these eventually resolve as well. There is no evidence that anaplasmosis can progress into a continuous, chronic illness such as PTLDS, and the pathogen responsible hasn't been shown to resist any antibiotics yet.

🅴❗ Alert

The standard antibiotic for anaplasmosis, doxycycline, is also the primary antibiotic recommended for Lyme disease. Therefore, if you have been diagnosed with anaplasmosis but have an undiagnosed infection with *B. burgdorferi*, or vice versa, your treatment will be effective and eliminate both pathogens.

Laboratory tests are used to confirm the doctor's diagnosis. In the early stages of the disease, the pathogen can be identified in white blood cells when looking at a blood sample under a microscope or it can be detected with a PCR test. Serologic tests are used but are typically negative in early disease because the immune system has not produced enough antibodies yet. For this reason, another blood sample, taken two to four weeks later, is usually tested, to show an increase in the number of antibodies to anaplasmosis compared to the early sample.

❓ Question

Can you get anaplasmosis more than once?
It appears the answer is no or, at the very least, it is highly unlikely. Patients who have had anaplasmosis seem to develop an immunity that keeps them protected against future infections.

Powassan Virus

In the spring of 2017, a number of news reports around the country were describing the appearance of a new tick-borne pathogen. This pathogen is called the Powassan virus, and it was linked to the deaths of several people in New York and Connecticut. It was also reportedly found in a five-month-old infant in Connecticut, who, fortunately, survived. According to the news reports, this "new" virus was being detected in up to 20 percent of ticks! The public was wisely told to be on alert for ticks and for symptoms of infection with this new tick-borne pathogen.

❓ Question

What is a virus and how is it different from a bacteria?
A virus is very different from any living organism. All living organisms on this planet, whether they are bacteria, fungi, or animals, are made up of living cells. Viruses aren't. The sole purpose of the existence of a virus is to infect cells in some host and force them to make more viruses. The cells very often die in the process. Viruses cannot exist on their own, which means they have to continuously infect new cells in order to survive.

Although at the time many reports made it appear that this was a new disease, the Powassan virus is not new at all. Scientists working in the field of tick-borne diseases were well aware of the Powassan virus for years, but it was relatively unknown to the public until the media flurry made it rather infamous in the first half of 2017. So, if the virus was known, why haven't you heard much about it until recently? The answer is rather simple. Human disease due to the Powassan virus is very rare, but, when it does occur, it is usually quite severe.

 Fact

The Powassan virus is part of a large group of viruses called flaviviruses. They are all typically transmitted either by mosquitoes or ticks. Other well-known flaviviruses that can cause disease in people are the West Nile virus, Zika virus, dengue virus, and yellow fever virus. All four are transmitted by mosquitoes.

The Powassan virus is named after the town of Powassan in Ontario, Canada, where the virus was first identified in the brain of a young boy who died of encephalitis in 1958. The virus can be transmitted by several different species of ticks. The majority of the people who have been bitten by ticks infected with the Powassan virus do not develop any disease. We know this because some people living in tick-endemic regions already have antibodies against the Powassan virus. This means they must have been infected in the past but never recall having any symptoms of the disease. In the smaller group of people where symptoms do develop, the disease can vary from mild to extremely severe and sometimes can be fatal.

Signs and Symptoms of Powassan Virus Disease

If you have been bitten by a tick infected with the Powassan virus, you may begin to feel ill any time between one and five weeks later. The illness typically begins with a fever. This is accompanied by a sore throat, headache, drowsiness, and disorientation. If the illness continues and the virus infects the central nervous system, it will lead to encephalitis, meningitis, or meningoencephalitis (inflammation of both the brain and the meninges). The symptoms of encephalitis include fever, vomiting, weakness, difficulty breathing and speaking, loss of coordination, confusion, and seizures. Parts of your body may have paralysis. Your eyes can be affected as well, resulting in the weakening of eye muscles. This can cause you to have an inability to keep your eyes in sync and difficulty in moving both eyes in every direction. You may also experience double or blurred vision.

 Alert

You may occasionally read a text that refers to either "septic" or "aseptic" meningitis. Septic refers to bacteria, while aseptic refers to lack of bacteria. Viruses are the main causes of aseptic meningitis.

Neurological disease due to the Powassan virus is a severe, potentially life-threatening illness, and nearly all patients with symptoms of Powassan virus disease develop the neurologic disease. Approximately 10 percent of patients who have symptoms of Powassan virus disease have died. About half of the patients who survived the severe illness continue to have long-lasting neurological problems, including paralysis in some parts of the body, loss of muscle, frequent headaches, and difficulty with memory.

Fact

In Europe, a somewhat similar virus is transmitted by the sheep tick called tick-borne encephalitis virus. As the name implies, it causes encephalitis, and approximately 10 percent of people infected with the virus die from the infection. This virus is more frequent in European ticks than the Powassan virus is in US ticks, and it causes about 10,000 cases of encephalitis each year throughout the European continent. Fortunately, a vaccine now exists that can prevent the disease.

Diagnosis and Treatment of Powassan Virus Disease

Diagnosing Powassan virus disease is not easy. The diagnosis is based on a combination of signs and symptoms and a positive result from laboratory tests of a blood sample obtained from the patient. First, a physician will examine you to see if you have any of the signs and symptoms associated with an infection with the Powassan virus. What they typically will look for is a high fever and evidence of neurological disease. If your symptoms fit the criteria, a sample will be taken and sent to a specialized laboratory for testing.

The two types of samples tested are usually blood and cerebrospinal fluid. Within the first week after you begin to show symptoms, the presence of the virus can be detected in these samples. In a laboratory, this can be done through growing the virus in a culture, although it can take days or weeks until enough viruses have been grown to conclusively identify the Powassan virus. A much quicker diagnosis can be achieved by performing a PCR test on either the blood or cerebrospinal fluid. Because a positive PCR result means that the virus is physically present, this is enough for a definitive diagnosis. If the specimen is taken later in the disease, the virus may not be present in either sample. In those cases, serologic tests are performed to find out if antibodies to the Powassan virus are present.

⊛ Essential

Cerebrospinal fluid is obtained by a process called lumbar puncture, although it is commonly referred to as a spinal tap. A spinal tap is frequently done on patients with a suspected infection of the central nervous system. During a spinal tap, a needle is carefully inserted into a region located in the back of the spine called the lumbar area, and the cerebrospinal fluid is drawn.

Unfortunately, there is no treatment that can cure a Powassan virus infection because antibiotics don't work. If you have a severe illness, you will need to be admitted to the hospital where supportive care will be provided. This typically consists of giving you intravenous fluids to keep you hydrated, ensuring proper breathing, and removing excess fluid from the brain that builds up as a result of the disease. Some patients have received high-dose corticosteroids, and all survived, though it is not yet clear if this treatment is beneficial or just a coincidence. Therefore, as with all tick-borne diseases, the primary advice is to ensure that you minimize contact with ticks.

⊛ Question

Why won't antibiotics work on the Powassan virus?
Antibiotics are used on organisms that are made up of cells and work by interfering with some important function in the cell. Because viruses are not cells, antibiotics have no effect on them.

Where and How Often Does Powassan Virus Disease Occur?

Historically, documented cases of neurologic disease caused by the Powassan virus are very rare. Between 1958, when the first case was reported, and 1998, there were only twenty-seven human cases reported in Canada and the United States. In a more recent period, between 2006 and 2015, sixty-eight confirmed cases of human neurologic disease caused by the Powassan virus were reported by the CDC. Three states had the majority of cases: Minnesota (twenty cases), Wisconsin (sixteen cases), and New York (sixteen cases). The disease was also reported in Massachusetts (eight cases), New Jersey (three cases), Maine (two cases), Virginia (one case), New Hampshire (one case), and Pennsylvania (one case). During this time, the number of cases reported annually ranged from just one in 2006 to twelve in both 2011 and 2013.

 Fact

Underreporting aside, if you live in the United States, you are more likely to be struck by lightning than to get encephalitis caused by the Powassan virus. In 2015, there were several hundred cases of lightning strikes, with twenty-seven deaths, as opposed to just six cases of Powassan virus disease.

All of these cases cluster in the northeastern and north-central parts of the United States, somewhat mirroring the distribution of Lyme disease. One substantial difference is that there have not been any reported cases of Powassan virus on the Pacific Coast, and so far, the virus has not been detected in ticks there. The increase of Powassan virus disease in the past two decades is likely due to two main factors. First, increased awareness of the Powassan virus may result in a higher likelihood of testing for the virus. Second, for some reason, the virus is more common in ticks now than it was thirty or forty years ago. Another possibility is that it's a combination of both of these factors that results in the increase in reporting of Powassan virus disease.

As with any tick-borne disease, the total number of cases of Powassan virus reported each year likely represents just a small portion of actual infections. Because patient specimens are not tested for the Powassan virus unless there is evidence of neurologic disease, very few patients actually get tested for it. In addition, mild neurologic disease in a Lyme disease–common region usually can be associated with neuroborreliosis, and hence, the patient is not tested for the Powassan virus. As an example of the lack of testing for this virus, not a single large commercial lab tested for the Powassan virus in 2008.

Vectors of the Powassan Virus

Two types of the Powassan virus are found in ticks. One is the "classical" virus that was identified in the 1950s. This virus is found primarily in two species of ticks, the squirrel tick, called *Ixodes marxi*, and the woodchuck tick, called *Ixodes cookei*. Although these ticks can bite people, they do so very rarely. Of these two, you're more likely to get infected from a woodchuck tick than a squirrel tick. Unlike blacklegged ticks, woodchuck ticks are typically not found on vegetation but rather in and around burrows of animals they feed on. Because of these feeding habits, these ticks rarely encounter people. Squirrel ticks also live near the homes of their namesakes, which means living in trees and other nests where humans rarely come in contact with them.

🄴 Alert

The woodchuck tick and the blacklegged tick are very similar in appearance and may be indistinguishable to the naked eye. Often, to tell them apart, you may have to observe them under a microscope.

The other type of the Powassan virus was first identified in 1997 in blacklegged ticks and was called the "deer tick virus." It was soon shown that the deer tick virus was a genetically different version of the Powassan virus. As you would expect, most recent cases of Powassan virus are caused by the virus found in black-legged ticks. However, a similar disease occurs after infection with either virus. Although some people still use the term "deer tick virus," this virus is usually now referred to as a type of the Powassan virus.

ⓔ❗ Alert

Both types of Powassan viruses are very similar to each another and it is not possible to tell them apart serologically. The only way to differentiate them is with a PCR test.

How Do Ticks Get Infected with the Powassan Virus?

Depending on the tick species, different animals serve as Powassan virus "reservoirs." The squirrel tick gets infected with the virus by feeding on infected squirrels, while woodchucks serve as the main reservoir for woodchuck ticks. On the other hand, blacklegged ticks get infected with the Powassan virus in the very same way these ticks get infected with *B. burgdorferi*: by feeding on infected white-footed mice, which, as is the case with *B. burgdorferi,* show no sign of disease upon infection with the Powassan virus. Once a tick is infected and reaches the adult stage, it can pass the virus to some of its eggs. This means some of the larvae may be infected with the Powassan virus even before feeding on an infected animal, unlike with Lyme disease.

One of the major differences between the Powassan virus and other pathogens you can get from blacklegged ticks is the length of time that a tick needs to attach before being able to transmit the virus. Remember, with Lyme disease, it can take anywhere from thirty-six to forty-eight hours until the bacteria is transmitted from the tick to your skin. In one study that examined ticks infected with the Powassan virus feeding on mice, it was observed that the virus could be transmitted in as little as fifteen minutes. This finding, if it holds true in people as well, has major implications for the potential of the virus to cause human disease. If only a short time is required for transmission of the Powassan virus, it would mean that the virus would be transmitted virtually every time an infected tick attaches. Rarely, if ever, are ticks spotted and removed almost immediately after attachment. Therefore, quick tick removal that would reduce the chances of acquiring *B. burgdorferi* and other agents would have little effect on Powassan virus transmission.

Frequency of Powassan Virus in Ticks

How frequently are ticks infected with the Powassan virus? And can infected ticks be found in all areas where blacklegged ticks are found? Unfortunately, there has not been nearly as much research on the Powassan virus as there has been on other tick-borne agents, primarily because of how rare it is. The data that is available shows that blacklegged ticks are infected with the Powassan virus much less frequently than with other pathogens. Typically, the virus will not be found in more than 3 percent of nymphs and 5 percent of adults. In most cases it's even lower, closer to 1 percent or not present at all. The exact geographic distribution of the Powassan virus is also not known right now, specifically whether or not it occurs outside of the somewhat limited areas where cases of this virus have been reported.

Borrelia miyamotoi

Borrelia miyamotoi is another pathogen that, in the past few years, has gotten substantial media exposure as a "new" tick-borne pathogen. However, here that description is quite justified. Although the Powassan virus has had a long history of causing disease in humans, *B. miyamotoi* has been associated with human disease only since 2011. As the *"Borrelia"* in the name suggests, *B. miyamotoi* is closely related genetically to *B. burgdorferi* and, when seen under a microscope, both bacteria look indistinguishable. However, the type of disease caused by *B. miyamotoi* as well as how often it occurs are both very different from Lyme disease.

 Fact

The infection with *B. miyamotoi* does not have a specific disease name. It is simply called *"Borrelia miyamotoi* disease."

B. miyamotoi was originally identified in 1995 in ticks and mice from Japan. Within the next ten years, it was subsequently shown to be present on both coasts of the United States in blacklegged and western blacklegged ticks. However, it received relatively little attention until 2011, when cases of human disease linked to *B. miyamotoi* were reported in Russia, the United States, Japan, and Europe. It is now recognized as yet another pathogen in the ever-growing spectrum of pathogens transmitted by the blacklegged and western blacklegged ticks.

Signs and Symptoms of *B. miyamotoi* Infection

Borrelia bacteria can cause two types of human diseases. One is Lyme disease and the other is called relapsing fever. The symptoms of these two diseases are very different. The main characteristic of relapsing fever is, as you could probably guess from the name, repeated episodes of fever, with some patients experiencing as many as six recurring episodes. In addition, the types of ticks are different for the two different diseases. Hard ticks transmit the *Borrelia* that cause Lyme disease, and soft ticks, as well as lice, transmit the bacteria that cause relapsing fever. *B. miyamotoi* is unusual in that it is a relapsing fever–type bacteria but is transmitted by a hard tick. Another difference is that *B. miyamotoi* can be passed from an adult female to her eggs, ensuring that some of the larvae will hatch infected with the bacteria, which has not been shown with *B. burgdorferi*.

The primary symptoms of *B. miyamotoi* disease are a fever that may exceed 104°F, fatigue, chills, nausea, muscle pain, and joint pain. In many of the initial symptoms, the disease does not differ very much from Lyme disease, and occasionally may be misdiagnosed as such. One major difference between the two diseases is that the EM rash is rarely seen in patients with *B. miyamotoi* disease, with only 8 percent of patients showing it in the one large study that has been done on *B. miyamotoi* disease.

ⓔ✓ Fact

In some cases of *B. miyamotoi* disease, the presence of an EM rash may be caused by a simultaneous infection with *B. burgdorferi*. It is possible that through the bite of a tick infected with both agents, you can get both diseases. A number of patients with a *B. miyamotoi* infection in Russia were shown to have had an EM rash due to concurrent Lyme disease.

As is characteristic for relapsing fever, if you have *B. miyamotoi* disease, you may experience episodes of a recurring fever. The initial fever will typically last about a week, followed by additional bouts of fever lasting one to five days. The time between the fevers can vary from at least two days to no more than seven. So far, the most episodes of recurring fever seen with *B. miyamotoi* disease has been three.

 Fact

Lyme disease, babesiosis, and anaplasmosis cannot be acquired through larval tick bites. However, because *B. miyamotoi* and the Powassan virus can be passed from the female adult tick to eggs and then subsequently to larvae, it is possible that either infection can be transmitted to you through the bite of a larval tick.

How Frequent Is *B. miyamotoi* Disease?

So far, *B. miyamotoi* disease is rare, with less than one hundred confirmed cases reported in the United States. It is likely that most infections don't show any symptoms. Other infections may be misdiagnosed as Lyme disease or other illnesses. Because of such infrequent occurrence, physicians and scientists still don't know the full scope of the disease associated with *B. miyamotoi*.

Essential

The white-footed mouse has been shown to be one of the main reservoir hosts for *B. miyamotoi*, which means this mouse can serve as a source of infection for all five agents carried by blacklegged ticks.

The areas in the United States where *B. miyamotoi* is present are also not well understood, mostly because of how rare it is. Very few studies looking at *B. miyamotoi* in ticks have been performed so far, and most of these have been limited to areas where cases of Lyme are the highest. In nymphal blacklegged ticks, *B. miyamotoi* can be found in anywhere from 0 to 10 percent, while in nymphal western blacklegged ticks, they vary from 0 to 15 percent.

Most of the time, the rates are much lower than 10 percent, usually between 1 and 5 percent. This lower prevalence in ticks partially explains why so few cases of *B. miyamotoi* infection have been identified so far.

 Fact

> *B. miyamotoi* is found in all the geographic regions where ticks associated with Lyme disease are found, including Europe and Asia, and *B. miyamotoi* disease is occasionally reported in countries on both continents.

Diagnosis and Treatment

B. miyamotoi infection lacks unique signs and symptoms, so diagnosis usually depends on diagnostic tests. Despite the fact that both *B. miyamotoi* and *B. burgdorferi* are genetically similar, the serologic tests for Lyme disease such as the two-tiered test are not helpful. Instead, a limited number of serologic tests more specific for *B. miyamotoi* have been developed. In addition, PCR tests are much more useful for *B. miyamotoi* disease than for Lyme disease. All relapsing fever *Borrelia*, including *B. miyamotoi*, tend to be present at a much higher concentration in the blood than *B. burgdorferi*, and therefore are much easier to detect. Several different PCR tests have been developed that are used to detect the presence of *B. miyamotoi* DNA in your blood. The serologic tests, along with the PCR tests, are available through a limited number of different commercial laboratories.

Infection with *B. miyamotoi* is treated similarly to an infection with *B. burgdorferi*. If you have an infection with *B. miyamotoi*, you will typically be prescribed a two- to four-week course of doxycycline. In children younger than nine as well as pregnant or nursing women, for whom doxycycline is not recommended,

the antibiotics amoxicillin and ceftriaxone have been successfully used.

Borrelia mayonii

As noted in Chapter 1, there is another species of *Borrelia*, called
Borrelia mayonii, that is transmitted by blacklegged ticks and can
cause Lyme disease in the United States. Very few cases of Lyme
disease caused by *B. mayonii* have been reported so far, all in Minnesota and Wisconsin. The Lyme disease caused by *B. mayonii*
appears similar to Lyme disease caused by *B. burgdorferi*, with
symptoms including a rash, fever, headache, and neck pain in
the early stages of disease and arthritis in later stages. Unlike *B.
burgdorferi*, however, *B. mayonii* infection is also associated with
nausea, vomiting, and other non–EM-like rashes. Another significant difference between *B. burgdorferi* and *B. mayonii* is that during infection, one hundred times more *B. mayonii* bacteria appear
in the blood than *B. burgdorferi*. This makes it easier to detect the
bacteria when testing blood by PCR, which, coincidently, was how
B. mayonii was initially discovered. The way doctors would diagnose Lyme disease caused by *B. mayonii* is probably the same as
for *B. burgdorferi*. Signs and symptoms may be used to diagnose
the early part of the disease, while the two-tier testing seems to
work in the later stages. PCR testing is also used. Treatment for
B. mayonii is the same as for *B. burgdorferi*, consisting of a two- to
four-week course of doxycycline.

🅴 Alert

So far, *B. mayonii* has only been found in the north-central United
States. Approximately 25,000 samples from patients living in forty-
three other states, including states in the Northeast and Mid-Atlantic
region, were tested for *B. mayonii* and all were negative.

Bartonellosis

Bartonella is a bacteria that causes infections collectively called bartonellosis. There has been a lot of confusion, disagreement, and controversy regarding whether *Bartonella* can be transmitted by ticks. Some doctors have reported a simultaneous infection with one species of *Bartonella*, *B. henselae*, in patients with Lyme disease. The presence of *Bartonella* DNA has frequently been detected in blacklegged ticks, as well as other ticks all over the world. This has led to the assumption that it is transmitted by ticks. This may be the case, but there is no definitive proof that this can actually happen. Although most people point to the presence of *Bartonella* DNA in ticks as proof that it is a tick-borne agent, you should be aware that finding the presence of DNA of an organism does not mean the organism is actually alive. Furthermore, it is not surprising to find *Bartonella* DNA in blacklegged ticks because of who they typically feed on. The majority of white-footed mice are infected with *Bartonella*, and since they serve as a primary blood meal for blacklegged ticks, it is very likely for traces of *Bartonella* DNA to remain inside ticks long after feeding on the mice. You can easily detect mouse DNA in a blacklegged tick as well. This DNA is simply material left over from the previous blood meal.

 Fact

By identifying the presence of DNA from different animals, you can determine which animals the tick fed on in previous life stages.

The best way to prove that a pathogen can be transmitted by ticks is by showing that ticks can be infected with that pathogen and then are able to pass the infection on to a new host during feeding. This has been done many times with all the pathogens known to be transmitted by blacklegged ticks. Until such an experiment is successfully done with *Bartonella*, it will remain unclear whether ticks can serve as a vector for this bacteria. Currently, the evidence that *Bartonella* can be tick-transmitted is very circumstantial and it is clear that more research is needed on this subject. However, because of a lack of clear, scientific proof, bartonellosis is not typically included on the list of tick-borne diseases in the United States.

Coinfections and the Severity of Lyme Disease

Because blacklegged ticks can be infected with so many different pathogens, it is possible that individual ticks can also be infected with more than one pathogen. In fact, pathogen coinfection has been well documented in blacklegged ticks as well as other ticks. For blacklegged ticks, the proportion of ticks that tend to be coinfected can vary dramatically, with geography being a major factor. The likelihood of a tick acquiring multiple pathogens depends on how frequently these pathogens are typically found in the area. Because tick-borne pathogens tend to be more common in areas where cases of Lyme disease are the highest, such as in the Northeast, these areas are also where coinfections in ticks are most frequent.

❓ Question

How does a single blacklegged tick get infected with multiple pathogens?

Blacklegged ticks typically get coinfected by feeding on a white-footed mouse that has multiple infections. For example, multiple nymphal ticks, some infected with *B. burgdorferi* and others with *B. microti*, feed on the same mouse. This mouse is then infected with both pathogens, and when an uninfected larval tick subsequently feeds on the same mouse, it will get infected with both pathogens. After it molts to the nymphal stage, this tick will be able to transmit both pathogens the next time it feeds.

Scientists acquire information about how often ticks are infected through a process called tick surveillance. This process consists of collecting ticks from different locations, and then testing them by PCR, either individually or in groups, for the presence of a particular pathogen. Then it is just simple math—divide the number of ticks infected with a pathogen by the number of ticks tested, and you get an answer on how frequently the pathogen can be found in ticks.

 Fact

Even if a pathogen has never been found in ticks within a particular area, you still cannot say that the risk of getting infected is zero. It is impossible to test all of the ticks, and there may be a very small proportion that were infected but were simply not tested.

The purpose of tick surveillance is to try to understand the level of risk residents of a particular community have for tick-borne diseases. The higher the frequency of a pathogen in ticks, the more likely that the disease will occur in that area. For example, *B. burgdorferi* is by far the most frequent pathogen in ticks, with about one in five nymphal ticks being infected. As a result, if you get bitten by a blacklegged tick nymph, there is an approximately one in five chance that you will get Lyme disease. However, in the very same area, another agent such as the Powassan virus may be absent in all of the ticks tested. This means that the risk of you getting the Powassan virus is potentially zero.

Coinfections in People

Because blacklegged ticks can be coinfected with multiple pathogens, what if you received a bite from a coinfected tick? Could you also simultaneously get more than one disease? The answer is yes, coinfections with tick-borne pathogens most certainly do occur. Unfortunately, even though coinfections may appear to be an important and fascinating topic, there have been relatively few reports that talk about how frequently they occur and whether they influence the severity of Lyme disease.

 Fact

In addition to getting bitten by a coinfected tick, you can get coin-fected with different pathogens by being bitten by multiple ticks, either together, or within a few days of each other.

Understanding how frequently a pathogen is found within an area can be very helpful for doctors in forming a potential diagnosis for a coinfection and in guiding their treatment. For example, in some counties in the Northeast, one out of every five blacklegged ticks may be infected with *B. microti*. If you reside in one of those counties, your doctor should be aware that a tick bite will expose you not only to Lyme disease, but also to babesiosis. If you go to the doctor with nonspecific signs, such as a fever, but don't have the obvious signs of Lyme disease, the doctor may be more likely to test you not just for Lyme disease, but for babesiosis as well, understanding that you might just have both.

Most Common Coinfections

The likelihood of acquiring a coinfection is directly related to the odds of coming across a coinfected blacklegged tick. The chances are much higher in the northeastern and north-central United States, where ticks have the highest infection rates in the country. Because *B. burgdorferi* is the most common pathogen in blacklegged ticks, followed by *B. microti* and *A. phagocytophilum*, the most frequent coinfections are typically *B. burgdorferi* with either *Babesia* or *Anaplasma*.

Fact

Recent research on Long Island, NY, showed how coinfections in ticks correlate with coinfections in people. On Long Island, about one out of every four blacklegged nymphs infected with *B. burgdorferi* can also be coinfected with *B. microti*. This would suggest that a high percentage of Lyme disease patients on Long Island may have babesiosis at the same time. When a group of Lyme disease patients from Long Island were also tested for babesiosis, about one quarter had antibodies to *B. microti*.

Frequency of Coinfections in People

How often are Lyme disease patients coinfected with another tick-borne illness? Unfortunately, that is not clear. Some studies have indicated that anywhere between 2 and 10 percent of Lyme disease patients may be coinfected with *Anaplasma*, while the frequency of coinfections of *B. burgdorferi* and *Babesia* can range from 2 to 40 percent.

Whether these numbers represent real coinfections or not is not clear. The way some scientists may define a coinfection affects how the rates of coinfections are reported. For example, many patients may have antibodies to more than one tick-borne agent. However, this does not mean that they were all coinfected. Although some may have been, others likely had these infections at different times. Remember, the presence of antibodies only indicates that an infection with a pathogen has occurred at some point, not when it occurred. To prove a coinfection, culturing both pathogens or confirming their presence by a PCR test would be needed, but these kinds of tests are rarely done.

Even though many doctors are aware that coinfections occur, an actual diagnosis of coinfections is very rarely reported. This is because of how tick-borne diseases are typically diagnosed and treated. If you have a tick-borne disease, there is a high probability that it will be Lyme disease, because it is the most common. If you have an EM rash, your doctor will prescribe you antibiotics right away. Even if your doctor recommends diagnostic testing, you will usually only be tested for Lyme disease. The standard antibiotic for Lyme disease, doxycycline, is also effective in treating any other tick-borne bacterial disease, such as anaplasmosis or *B. miyamotoi* disease, so even if you were coinfected with these pathogens, you will likely never know and neither will your doctor.

Coinfections become a bigger problem if you have nonbacterial agents such as *B. microti* or the Powassan virus. Here doxycycline treatment would not eliminate the coinfection because antibiotics don't work on these agents. Although *B. burgdorferi* may be gone, it would appear that the antibiotic treatment did not work because the presence of the coinfecting agent would cause continuing symptoms. In these cases, your doctor could very well begin to suspect a coinfection and have your sample tested for other pathogens.

Disease Severity Due to Coinfections

Unfortunately, not much is known about how coinfections affect the severity of Lyme disease because very few studies have investigated this. You could presume that by being infected with two different pathogens at the same time you would have two different diseases, and therefore have much more severe symptoms. However, that might not always be the case.

Some studies have shown that if you have Lyme disease and babesiosis at the same time, you may have more symptoms that last for a longer period of time than you would if you had Lyme disease alone. You may also be more likely to have some babesiosis-like disease manifestations, including anemia, low platelet count, or an enlarged spleen. However, this may occur more often in older patients because these are the patients who are more likely to have symptoms of babesiosis. It is possible that in most younger patients, the combined symptoms of Lyme disease and babesiosis may not be very different from those of Lyme disease alone.

Some patients with a coinfection with *B. burgdorferi* and *Anaplasma* have also reported an increased number of symptoms. However, other patients haven't. And because *B. miyamotoi* and Powassan virus infections are so rare, there is nothing known about what happens to the severity of Lyme disease if you are coinfected with either of these two agents. Because there have been so few studies on coinfections with tick-borne agents in general, scientists have a very limited understanding of this phenomenon.

Summary

Besides *B. burgdorferi*, there are a number of other pathogens that can be transmitted by blacklegged ticks. In addition to Lyme disease, blacklegged ticks can transmit other pathogens that cause four other diseases, including babesiosis, anaplasmosis, Powassan virus disease, and *Borrelia miyamotoi* disease. There is also another *Borrelia*, called *Borrelia mayonii*, that can cause Lyme disease in the upper-central region of the United States. These coinfections mostly occur from nymphal tick bites in the northeastern and upper-central areas of the United States. They are all less common than Lyme disease.

Out of these four diseases, ticks are most frequently infected with *Babesia microti* and *Anaplasma phagocytophilum*, which are the pathogens that cause babesiosis and anaplasmosis. Both diseases are reported in about 1,500 people every year, the majority of whom are over 40 years old. In addition to tick bites, both diseases can also be acquired through blood transfusions.

Diseases caused by *B. miyamotoi* and the Powassan virus are rarely diagnosed, mainly because both pathogens are rarely found in ticks. *B. miyamotoi* disease is caused by a spirochete similar to *B. burgdorferi* but causes a different disease called relapsing fever. Infections with the Powassan virus can cause a very severe disease when the virus infects the brain. About one out of every ten people who have Powassan virus disease die from it. Because it is a virus, therapy used for other diseases will not work, and there is no known cure for a Powassan virus infection. Unlike other pathogens transmitted by the blacklegged tick, both *B. miyamotoi* and Powassan virus can be passed from the adult tick female to her eggs and subsequently to larvae. This means both pathogens can be transmitted by the bites of larval ticks, unlike with Lyme disease. White-footed mice are the main animal hosts for all of the pathogens transmitted by blacklegged ticks, and they can sometimes be infected with multiple pathogens at the same time. Ticks get coinfected with multiple pathogens when they feed on these mice and can then pass multiple infections to people. Babesiosis and anaplasmosis are the most frequent coinfections in patients with Lyme disease, and in some instances, coinfection can increase the severity of Lyme disease.

CHAPTER 9

Research for the Future

As you approach the end of this book, you may find yourself wondering what the outlook is for the future as it pertains to Lyme disease. Are scientists working on anything significant that will hopefully reduce the frequency of Lyme disease or perhaps prevent it altogether? Is there hope for an improvement in how the disease is diagnosed and treated? You will be relieved to find out that many scientists are indeed currently working on all of these different aspects of Lyme disease. This chapter will review some of the innovative ways scientists are trying to approach the problem of Lyme disease and what impact these studies will have for the future.

Ecological Prevention

What is the best way to avoid Lyme disease? The simplest answer is to avoid getting bitten by ticks. Scientists are always looking for different ways within communities to lower the chance of people getting bitten by limiting their exposure to *B. burgdorferi*. In these studies, scientists are trying to change the life cycle of the bacteria, which eventually will reduce the likelihood of people getting Lyme disease. Over the past thirty-five years, a number of ecological prevention studies have focused on examining whether it is possible to decrease the number of, or perhaps even eliminate, blacklegged ticks in the environment. The thinking is quite simple: by reducing the number of ticks that are present in your community, you are much less likely to encounter them and get bitten. Fewer tick bites result in less Lyme disease.

The best way to reduce the number of ticks in residential areas is to spray acaricides, which are a form of a pesticide geared more toward eliminating ticks and mites. Like normal pesticides, they are generally sprayed on vegetation where ticks are normally found. A single application of an acaricide can reduce the number of blacklegged nymphs between 60 to 100 percent within residential properties. The main problem with acaricides, however, is that they can be toxic, which means they should be applied as rarely as possible. Because of unease over potential health problems, some people may be hesitant to use them.

Deer Control

Besides spraying acaricides, scientists have explored other ways to control tick populations, primarily through interfering with the normal life cycle of the blacklegged tick. One way to do this is by removing the animal hosts that the blacklegged ticks need to survive. If the ticks don't have these essential hosts to feed on, they can't complete their life cycle. This would mean fewer ticks laying eggs, which would obviously lead to fewer ticks in future generations.

As discussed in Chapter 2, deer are essential hosts for blacklegged tick adults. A large increase in the numbers of deer in the twentieth century likely had a direct role in the upsurge in the population of blacklegged ticks. It would also make sense if the opposite were true. By eliminating deer, the population of the blacklegged ticks should decline. However, the effects are not that simple. Instead, the impact on the tick population can vary, depending on whether the deer are completely or only partially eliminated. Also, whether or not this really reduces the rate of Lyme disease is still not clear.

Several studies in the Northeast have examined what happens to tick populations when the number of deer are reduced. As we mentioned in Chapter 2, on an island off the coast of Maine called Monhegan Island, scientists found that eliminating deer was extremely helpful in reducing the number of ticks. Three years after all deer were purged, not a single larval or nymphal blacklegged tick could be found. This showed that a complete removal of all deer within an area would eliminate the blacklegged tick populations and the chances of you getting Lyme disease.

❓ Question

How are these deer control studies run?
After an area is chosen for a study, the deer are hunted to reduce the population. Once the deer population decreases, scientists collect ticks over the next few years, counting how many ticks they find each season. They then compare the numbers to see if the number of ticks has gone down.

However, the results of other studies that looked at the effects on ticks after the deer population is reduced, but not eliminated, were somewhat mixed. In a few other studies, the deer population at sites in Massachusetts, Connecticut, and New Jersey was reduced to one fifth their original number or less. In most areas, the number of nymphal blacklegged ticks went down over the next few years as well. In one study, though, the tick population didn't go down at all. Although the findings were not unanimous, it does look like reducing the number of deer around an area helps control the tick population as well.

The results of these studies were promising, but there were a few things that weren't taken into account. The studies were mostly focused on the environmental aspects and were performed in areas with very few people. This means we don't know for sure that reducing the number of ticks would also reduce the number of Lyme disease diagnoses in an area. In addition, most of the studies were done in enclosed settings, such as an island, so no deer could wander into site, as would normally happen in nature. There's a concern that even if the deer population of an area were reduced, over time, deer from other areas would migrate in. This would eventually lead to the number of ticks returning to normal levels.

Other studies have looked at the possibility of killing ticks while they feed on deer. Treating deer with an acaricide should theoretically kill any feeding ticks. If enough deer were treated, then perhaps enough ticks would be killed and fewer ticks would be seen in subsequent years. One of the ways this idea was tested was by using a device called a "4-poster deer treatment bait station." This device has two rollers with acaricide on them on either side of a bin filled with corn kernels. The way it's set up, in order to get the corn, the deer has to be in contact with the rollers. As the deer feeds, the rollers apply the acaricide to the head, neck, and ears of the deer. When the deer grooms itself, it spreads the acaricide to the rest of the body.

After some studies were done in the Northeast, it was shown to be a pretty effective way to reduce the number of blacklegged ticks. In some areas, nearly every single tick was eliminated. Even better, this method is safer for people and more environmentally friendly than acaricide spraying. One thing that does remain unclear, however, is the long-term effects of the acaricide on the deer itself.

White-Footed Mouse Control

Alternatively, reducing the number of *B. burgdorferi*-infected ticks should have the same effect as reducing the total number of ticks in the environment. Although tick bites may be inevitable, if the ticks you are exposed to are rarely infected, the chances of you getting Lyme disease will be much lower. To accomplish this, some scientists have looked at the mice that act as a reservoir for *B. burgdorferi* as a potential way for Lyme disease to be controlled. Obviously, mice control in the wild is not possible. Instead, scientists focused on ways they could minimize the numbers of mice that were infected with *B. burgdorferi*. For example, what if you vaccinate mice against *B. burgdorferi*? Would that result in a reduction of *B. burgdorferi*-infected ticks? And even if it did, how could you possibly vaccinate mice out in the wild?

This interesting approach was investigated by a group of scientists who used a safe oral vaccine that was mixed with food and fed to wild mice to immunize them against the bacteria. After that, any infected tick that fed on an immunized mouse wouldn't be able to transmit the infection. And because the mouse could not be infected, any uninfected tick that also fed on this mouse would not get infected either. If enough mice were immunized, fewer ticks would be able to pass on the bacteria or get it passed on to them, lowering the overall number of infected ticks in the wild.

Over the course of five years, ticks were collected near where the scientists fed the vaccine to the mice. After two years, there were about 25 percent fewer infected ticks in the areas around the feeding sites and after five years, there were 75 percent fewer infected ticks. A long-term program using this method put in place around residential areas could result in fewer people with Lyme disease.

Another study did this with a slight spin on it. Instead of vaccinating the mice against *B. burgdorferi*, the antibiotic doxycycline was added to the food for the mice. By eating the antibiotic, any mice that were infected with *B. burgdorferi* would be cured of the infection. Because they weren't infected with the bacteria anymore, they wouldn't be able to infect any ticks. The study showed that this is exactly what happened—with fewer infected mice, there were fewer infected ticks to spread Lyme disease.

Other Methods

Scientists are exploring other ecological prevention methods. One particularly interesting study that is currently underway is using genetic manipulation to create white-footed mice that are immune to *B. burgdorferi*. Using a new method called CRISPR (clustered regularly interspaced short palindromic repeats), which allows scientists to change the genes of any organism, the scientists involved with the project believe that they could genetically modify mice into being resistant to infection, and they could then pass this resistance on to their offspring. First, the scientists would identify the genes in mice that are responsible for creating antibodies against *B. burgdorferi*. Once the genes are found, they would be placed into the reproductive cells of other mice. Those mice would then pass them, along with the immunity they provide, onto all of their offspring. These genetically altered mice will be first released on islands, which makes it easier for scientists to observe whether these mice decrease the rates of infected ticks in an isolated area without other mice coming in and out.

Potential for Future Use

Many of these different studies appear promising in controlling tick populations. But they face some obstacles before they can be used more frequently, such as costs or concerns over pesticide use. There are also some concerns about the assumption that fewer ticks mean fewer cases of Lyme disease. Though that assumption may appear obvious, it may not necessarily be true. There have been studies using pesticides that showed declines in tick populations, but not in tick bites. Scientists are still not sure why that would happen, so more work needs to be done before we can conclusively say that reducing the number of ticks will lower the frequency of Lyme disease.

Diagnostic Improvements

One of the major goals of scientists working in the field of Lyme disease is a better diagnostic test than the currently used two-tiered test. As discussed in Chapter 5, many research groups have developed or are in the process of developing new tests for Lyme disease. Over the past decade, a wide variety of different tests have been developed that appear to improve upon the two-tiered test. It seems that creating a better test is not the biggest problem. Instead, ensuring that it is universally available, easy to use, and relatively inexpensive are the biggest challenges. Currently, the two-tiered test, despite its shortcomings, fulfills all of these criteria.

Improved Serologic Tests

One aspect of serologic testing that could be improved is developing more specific tests. As a reminder, serologic tests, such as the two-tiered ELISA and Western blot, test for antibodies that are made by your immune system in response to a pathogen rather than the pathogen itself. One of the main drawbacks with the ELISA used in the two-tiered test is that it uses all of the proteins of *B. burgdorferi*, some of which are also found on other bacteria, as targets for antibodies. If the sample had antibodies made to fight against a different pathogen that had the same type of protein as *B. burgdorferi*, it would trigger the test and be a false positive. A better ELISA test would consist of only the proteins from *B. burgdorferi* that your immune system targets, particularly early on in the infection. This would create a test that is very sensitive and very specific to *B. burgdorferi*. In fact, that is the main achievement of the C6 ELISA, which is based on a small fragment of a single *B. burgdorferi* protein. And adding a few more targets on top of the C6 would improve the sensitivity of the test even more.

Considerable efforts have been devoted by scientists to identify *B. burgdorferi* proteins that our immune system recognizes early on during the infection. By now, the majority of them are known. The serologic tests that are currently being developed use a combination of these proteins as targets. This is probably the best way to create tests that are more specific and sensitive than the two-tiered test. Some of these tests have already started to be more widely used in the clinical laboratories that perform testing for Lyme disease. Several others have been initially tested and show great promise as well. In the end, it may not be very long until the two-tiered test is supplanted by more effective tests.

Next-Generation Sequencing

As mentioned in Chapter 5, next-generation sequencing (also called high-throughput sequencing) is a new way to diagnose Lyme disease, with the ability to identify the DNA of every organism in a sample. Although it is only used by a few labs at this time, it is being used more and more in recent years. Unfortunately, right now the costs are still very high but inevitably they will go down, and it's very likely that within the next five to ten years, many clinical labs will be able to use this method for diagnosis of early disease. A major advantage of next-generation sequencing over the standard PCR tests currently in use is that it can identify all infectious agents in a sample, not just *B. burgdorferi*, so it would diagnose any coinfections present as well as Lyme disease.

In addition to its use in diagnosis, several groups are using next-generation sequencing to examine all the different microbes that can be found in ticks. Despite our best efforts, we still don't know all the infectious agents that could cause potential coinfections that may be present in ticks. It seems almost every year a new tick-borne pathogen suddenly appears, whether it's a virus such as the Heartland virus or a new Lyme disease bacteria such as *B. mayonii*.

Because next-generation sequencing can detect and identify all of the genetic signatures in a sample, it is perfect for discovering new potential pathogens. For example, if you were testing a DNA sample from a single tick and it contained fifty different microbes, next-generation sequencing would likely be able to identify all of them. Using this method to test different species of ticks from different geographic areas would allow scientists to discover new pathogens even before people get infected. Instead of a brand-new pathogen appearing out of nowhere and causing disease, it can be identified first in ticks and diagnostic tests; cures can be created. This way, doctors and scientists can be ready if and when the disease emerges into the population at large. An example of the power of this platform is the fact that until recently, the Powassan virus was the only virus that was known to be in blacklegged ticks. Using next-generation sequencing, scientists were able to identify more than twenty others. Now, it is unlikely that most of these cause disease, but some may. This lets scientists get a head start on identifying any of these potentially disease-causing viruses.

Multiplex Tests

One problem with both the molecular and serologic diagnostic tests out there right now is that they only test for one disease at a time. But as we now know from Chapter 8, blacklegged ticks can transmit five or more infectious agents and ticks can occasionally be coinfected with more than one. If you have Lyme disease, there is always a risk that you may have acquired a coinfection as well. It is important that patients who think they have any tick-borne disease get tested for the wide range of agents that they may have been exposed to. Unfortunately, that's not often done. Tests for other agents, if they're even available, are done separately, which can be both time consuming and very costly. A typical test for Lyme disease may cost $200. If you want to test for babesiosis, the cost may be another $200. For anaplasmosis, another $200, and so on. At the end of the day, the cost of the testing can easily reach $1,000.

One way to minimize both the labor and the cost of testing is by using multiplex tests. Multiplex tests check for more than one agent at a time. In the past decade, PCR is the one diagnostic platform where multiplex tests have been increasingly used instead of single-agent tests. A number of multiplex PCR tests have been developed by different research groups and clinical labs. They have been successfully used for testing ticks to obtain more accurate estimates of how often ticks are coinfected with different pathogens. They are also being used more frequently in testing samples from people with possible tick-borne illnesses. Because PCR is currently the most sensitive test and is most useful for detecting Lyme disease in its early stage, more widespread use of multiplex PCR testing will be very useful for obtaining a much more accurate diagnosis and should lessen the number of undiagnosed infections or coinfections.

Multiplex serologic tests are much more difficult to develop. Because antibodies aren't always specific to one agent, creating tests that are specific to each pathogen and then running them together is extremely difficult. The good news is that substantial progress has been made in this area. In fact, some tests have proven this is at least feasible, with some being able to tell the difference between antibodies for up to five or more pathogens in a single test. Although these aren't yet ready for clinical use, the fact that these tests have at least been developed presents hope that multiplex serologic tests will be available to the public in the not too distant future.

Xenodiagnosis

Xenodiagnosis is a process that has recently been used to figure out whether there are any live bacteria in patients with PTLDS. This could help solve the controversy surrounding the idea that some live bacteria can survive after antibiotic treatments, one of the main beliefs of people with chronic Lyme disease. Although PCR tests can detect the presence of bacterial DNA, they can't tell the difference between live or dead bacteria. Trying to culture the bacteria has not worked, so some scientists have turned to xenodiagnosis to help solve this mystery.

In xenodiagnosis, volunteer patients with PTLDS allow larval blacklegged ticks to feed on them. The ticks that are used for this are raised in a lab so the scientists know for sure that they don't yet have the *B. burgdorferi* bacteria. After the ticks finish their feeding, the scientists check to see whether they have any of the bacteria inside their gut. The rationale is that if any live bacteria really are in the blood of a patient with PTLDS, they may be acquired by the ticks during the feeding. Finding the bacteria in the larval tick is just the first step. At this point, any bacteria that is present may not necessarily be alive. However, if these ticks then molted to become nymphs and were able to transfer the bacteria to a clean lab mouse, it would conclusively show that there were indeed live bacteria in the patient with PTLDS. Some studies looking into this have just begun and have not yielded any conclusive results yet. If they are successful, they may open up a whole new area of research as well as alter the way many scientists view PTLDS.

 Fact

Xenodiagnosis is also used as a diagnostic tool for a disease called Chagas disease, which occurs in Central and South America. Chagas disease is a parasitic disease transmitted by large bugs called kissing or assassin bugs. To diagnose patients, uninfected bugs are allowed to feed on them before being examined for the presence of parasites.

Other Diagnostic Methods

The rapid technological advances that have occurred in the past fifteen years have opened the door to the possibility of exploring some tests with new diagnostic techniques, such as accurately measuring different changes in the body that occur as a result of an infection. As mentioned in Chapter 5, some groups have used the study of metabolomics to identify minute biochemical changes in the blood of patients soon after they are infected with *B. burgdorferi*. These changes occur only in patients with Lyme disease, and in the future, may be the basis for a diagnostic test that could potentially identify the presence of *B. burgdorferi* earlier than any molecular or serologic test. In addition, scientists are now exploring metabolomics to identify biochemical changes that occur after an infection with other tick-borne pathogens. These changes, once identified, can then be used not only for diagnosis, but also to differentiate among different diseases. For example, scientists have recently identified the different biochemical changes between patients with STARI and Lyme disease. Whereas it may be difficult for a doctor to distinguish between a STARI and Lyme disease rash, metabolomic analysis of biochemical changes when the rash first appears can quickly identify the disease.

Other new platforms have the ability to look for changes in cytokines, which are small proteins that our cells use to send signals to other cells. During infection, a large number of cytokines are produced by our body to initiate a wide variety of events, including inflammation. Scientists are looking to see whether there are any cytokines that can be used as a predictor of disease. For example, it has been shown that when someone gets neuroborreliosis, the levels of one specific cytokine increase, which is important because there is no current diagnostic test that can identify this condition. By testing for this cytokine, perhaps patients with neuroborreliosis can be more easily identified.

Effective Treatment

Is Lyme disease treatment effective? To a large extent, it is. Can it be improved? Certainly. This is an area where much more research needs to be done. All groups, even ones holding drastically different views on the existence of chronic Lyme disease, do agree that antibiotic treatment is the most effective way to eliminate a *B. burgdorferi* infection. But that's where the agreement ends.

Unfortunately, there have been relatively few studies that have compared how well different antibiotics can prevent the growth of *B. burgdorferi*. Scientists also don't know exactly what the best amount of time is for people taking these drugs, especially with different age groups. Because there are so many questions regarding the proper treatment, more studies are clearly needed. These studies need to be well-designed trials that clearly show the benefit, or lack thereof, of any medication, pharmaceutical or otherwise.

In particular, the question of how long the treatment should last needs to be addressed. It is rather distressing that in this day and age, with the vast advances in technology, this issue still can't be clearly resolved. Unless it's shown that there are live bacteria still hanging around posttreatment, the current recommended treatments for each of the stages of Lyme disease will likely not change in the near future. As a result, the argument surrounding a long-term antibiotic treatment will also likely not change. However, even if you do have a persistent, "incurable" infection, being on antibiotics at all times is not the answer because the risks to your health will be too extreme. So if not antibiotics, then what? That's the problem. Some of the alternative treatments that were described in Chapter 6 are very sketchy and are likely not the answer either. Is integrative medicine the answer? Perhaps. At the end of the day, anything that reduces your symptoms should be considered, as long as it has been shown to be safe and will not further damage your health.

Lyme Disease Vaccination

The best way to avoid the unpleasantness of Lyme disease is to prevent the infection from occurring in the first place. Getting vaccinated would provide a safety net, even if you happen to get bitten by infected ticks. In Chapter 7, you learned about the original Lyme vaccine LYMErix and its quick fall from grace. Since LYMErix, no new vaccines have been introduced to the market. This is unfortunate, as the number of Lyme disease cases in the United States has only grown during that time and a vaccine for Lyme disease is sorely needed. Fortunately, scientists have continued to search for Lyme disease vaccines. Some of these prospective vaccines have used the same, but slightly modified, target as LYMErix, while others have focused on alternative proteins that may be more effective in providing protection from Lyme disease.

🅔 Alert

The LYMErix vaccine worked in a different way than typical vaccines. Instead of building up your immune system to fight back against *B. burgdorferi* once it was inside you, it would attack the bacteria while it was still inside a tick that was feeding on you. When your blood reached the tick's gut, the antibodies produced because of the vaccine would help kill the bacteria inside the tick. Thus, the bacteria never had a chance to actually enter your body.

OspA Vaccine

As discussed in Chapter 7, one of the problems with the LYMErix vaccine was the possibility that a small part of the OspA protein that was being used as the target was similar to a small fragment of a human protein. This was suspected to be a possible cause of the autoimmunity problem as well as the adverse symptoms reported by some people immunized with the vaccine. Another weakness of the vaccine was the fact that it only targeted a type of *B. burgdorferi* OspA that was found exclusively in the United States. Therefore, the vaccine would not protect people infected in Europe, where other species of *Borrelia* are more likely to cause Lyme disease.

Despite the withdrawal of the original vaccine, at the end of the day, it did work at protecting against Lyme disease. Since that time, various groups have tried to alter the original vaccine and eliminate these problems. For example, different companies have been developing vaccines that combine all the different types of OspA that are present in *Borrelia* in both the United States and Europe. Producing a vaccine that has universal applications is more financially sound for a manufacturer, ensuring that it remains on the market. These vaccines are also missing the part of the protein that was similar to the human protein, meaning they shouldn't lead to autoimmunity, and this removes the main controversial aspect of the vaccine. This vaccine appears to have promise. A pharmaceutical company in Europe has in fact already begun clinical trials and is testing this vaccine in Europe and the United States.

🅔❗ Alert

Despite the earlier theory that the IFA-1-like fragment that is present on OspA can trigger autoimmunity, this association has been since disproven. However, to avoid any controversies, any new OspA-based vaccines omit this part in the vaccine.

OspC Vaccine

Another approach for Lyme disease vaccine development is to target a protein other than OspA. A number of different *B. burgdorferi* proteins have been explored as potential targets. One of these is known as OspC. OspC is an essential protein needed for *B. burgdorferi* to establish an infection immediately after it's transmitted from the tick. It is also a major target of human antibodies early in the infection, potentially making OspC an ideal vaccine target. However, using OspC for a target in a vaccine is not easy. Because there are so many strains, *B. burgdorferi* has vast genetic diversity, a major problem when designing a vaccine against it. This is especially true for OspC.

B. burgdorferi can have over twenty different types of OspC, and immunity against one type does not necessarily mean immunity against another type. To create an effective vaccine, scientists need to consider all the different variants that may be present in ticks. This adds another layer of difficulty because it is challenging enough to create an effective vaccine to just one type. One group has developed such a vaccine, which contains fragments of several different OspC types mixed together. If you were to be immunized with this vaccine, you should become immune to all the different types. Although it looks promising from a medical perspective, it remains to be seen if this vaccine will eventually progress into larger trials.

Other groups have explored using other *B. burgdorferi* protein as vaccine targets. The majority of these potential vaccines are still in the prototype stages and are not ready for clinical trial testing. Several groups have also explored a method of mixing several different *Borrelia* proteins together in order to make a stronger vaccine. One such vaccine, using three different proteins, was developed, and in mice studies was more effective than using only a single protein. Unfortunately, more tests have not been done yet.

Vaccination Against Other Tick-Borne Pathogens

Lyme disease is just one of the diseases that can be acquired from a bite of the blacklegged tick. Although creating an effective vaccine for Lyme disease is the biggest priority, vaccines against other agents are needed as well. Unfortunately, there are no currently available vaccines for any of the other tick-borne pathogens present in the United States. Research groups are investigating the likelihood of creating vaccines against these agents though they are still far away from any large-scale clinical trials in humans. This doesn't mean that it will not happen, but it's more likely that a new Lyme disease vaccine will be available before a vaccine for any of the other tick-borne pathogens in the United States. However, one appealing possibility is the potential for creating a vaccine that will contain parts of several tick-borne agents. Such a vaccine, in theory, would protect against not just Lyme disease, but perhaps against anaplasmosis and babesiosis as well, thus providing immunity against potential coinfections. The possibility of such vaccines is currently being investigated.

Tick Protein Vaccines

Some groups working on Lyme disease vaccines have proposed using a very interesting and altogether different approach. Instead of using *B. burgdorferi* proteins to vaccinate against Lyme disease, these groups are focusing on the development of anti-tick vaccines, where the person would have immunity to the tick and not the bacteria. However, the vaccine would essentially perform the same function with the same outcome: prevention of the transmission of *B. burgdorferi* from the tick vector to the animal host.

How would such a vaccine work? The basis of anti-tick vaccines is the development of something called "tick immunity." Some animals, after receiving several bites from the same species of tick, develop antibodies to the proteins that are present in the tick saliva. When that same type of tick tries to feed on this animal again, it's instead killed by the immune system of the animal. Other times, even if the tick is not killed, the immune response interferes and prevents the tick from feeding so it can't pass along any bacteria or viruses.

To make an anti-tick vaccine, scientists would need to identify suitable saliva proteins of the blacklegged tick that could serve as targets for the vaccine. A number of these tick saliva proteins have already been identified and are being studied as potential vaccine targets. After receiving the vaccine, the person would develop antibodies to the tick saliva. Then, if a blacklegged tick attempted to feed on that person, the tick would either be rejected and fall off or it would be killed outright. An added benefit of such a vaccine is that it would prevent the transmission of all tick-borne pathogens, not only *B. burgdorferi*. Therefore, in the long run, anti-tick vaccines may prove to be even better than vaccines targeting specific agents. Progress with these types of vaccines is being made in both the United States and in Europe, and it would not be surprising if they are ready for trials within the next five years or so.

Insights Into the Disease

Every symptom of Lyme disease that you develop during the course of the illness connects to something that *B. burgdorferi* is doing in your body. Understanding these connections is the focus of a large number of current scientific studies. Learning more about how *B. burgdorferi* causes disease is important in improving diagnosis and treatment. One way this is being done is by using animals, which enables the study of different aspects of Lyme disease.

Animal Models of Lyme Disease

Through interaction with patients, doctors and researchers can learn a lot about what *B. burgdorferi* may be doing to your body. As you can imagine, however, they don't know *exactly* what is happening; it's a bit of educated guesswork. The damage that *B. burgdorferi* actually inflicts on the body is difficult to investigate. For example, questions such as "What happens to the heart when it is invaded by *B. burgdorferi*?" or "Can you really find *B. burgdorferi* in the brain?" are difficult to answer because such invasive studies are obviously not possible in people. So how do we know the extent of the damage *B. burgdorferi* can actually inflict? Through studies with animals.

In order to learn more about the extent of a disease, scientists try to replicate it in a susceptible animal. The goal is to find an animal that, when infected by the pathogen, will exhibit the signs and symptoms that are similar to a human infection. This is called an "animal model" of a disease. In an animal model, scientists can investigate how the disease progresses in ways they never could otherwise.

Fact

There are many genetically different types of lab mice. Interestingly, the signs of Lyme disease in laboratory mice can also differ depending on which type is used for experiments. For instance, while some strains of mice get arthritis, others do not. This shows the importance of host genetics in the ability to prevent severe disease.

For the past 30 years or so, mice have been used as animal models for Lyme disease. Although white-footed mice and other rodents that are infected by *B. burgdorferi* in the wild do not show signs of any disease, some types of laboratory mice have been shown to develop arthritis and carditis after being infected with the bacteria. By using these mice, scientists have learned a great deal about the pathology of Lyme disease. For example, the reason we know that *B. burgdorferi* can cause heart block is by studying this condition in *B. burgdorferi*-infected mice. We also know that some strains of *B. burgdorferi* tend to cause a more severe infection than others by studying the severity of the disease that these strains cause in mice.

Fact

The reason scientists believe it takes about thirty-six to forty-eight hours to get Lyme disease is that this is how long it takes for mice to get infected with *B. burgdorferi* in various studies. It is presumed that a similar amount of time is needed for human infection, but whether that is in fact true is not 100 percent certain because such studies cannot be done in people.

Studies using animals have many drawbacks as well. Mice, obviously, are not humans, and their physiology is different from ours. The way Lyme disease progresses in a mouse may be different from how it progresses in a human being. Although mice develop arthritis and carditis, they do not develop an EM rash or any neurologic symptoms. Thus, scientists cannot learn anything about neuroborreliosis from a mouse animal model. To learn about neuroborreliosis, scientists have used other animal models, such as dogs or rhesus monkeys. Dogs develop arthritis and facial palsies after being infected with *B. burgdorferi*. Rhesus monkeys, one of the closest animals to humans genetically and physiologically, can develop an EM rash, neuroborreliosis, and arthritis after infection. However, because of higher costs and a substantial increase in the difficulty of the work, these animals are used much less frequently in studies than mice.

Persistence of *B. burgdorferi* after Antibiotic Treatment

One way animal models have had a huge impact on our understanding of Lyme disease has been to show that some *B. burgdorferi* could survive in a host even after antibiotic treatment. For many years, there was a widely held view that a standard antibiotic regimen would be successful in completely clearing an infection of *B. burgdorferi*. As a result, scientists and doctors believed that any signs and symptoms that appeared after the treatment could not have been caused by an active infection, but were instead triggered by other unknown factors. In the last fifteen years, however, several studies using animal models have shown that this view is most likely incorrect.

B. burgdorferi has been shown to establish a persistent infection in many different hosts. In these hosts, the bacteria sometimes cannot be completely cleared from the body for a very long time. *B. burgdorferi* can cause a persistent infection in mice, rats, hamsters, gerbils, guinea pigs, pigs, dogs, and monkeys and has occasionally caused a persistent infection in people. In one case, live *B. burgdorferi* was cultured from a skin sample taken from a patient ten years after the initial infection.

Once it was determined that these bacteria can establish a long-term infection in animals, scientists then looked at animal models to see whether it could continue even after treatment with antibiotics. It turns out *B. burgdorferi* DNA could be detected in mice, dogs, and even rhesus monkeys after antibiotic treatments had been completed. However, it also appears that the persistent bacteria tend to be quite different from the typical *B. burgdorferi*, and most important, they appear to be unable to cause disease. However, their sheer existence is intriguing to everyone studying Lyme disease.

So, can this also occur in people? Unfortunately, that is not yet clear. *B. burgdorferi* DNA can be detected in synovial fluid, which is the fluid present in the joints, for months after the initiation of antibiotic therapy. However, these are rare events, and in most cases live bacteria, or any bacteria at all, cannot be shown. In addition, even if the bacterial DNA is present, it doesn't necessarily mean that live bacteria are present. Thus, although it is a focus of intense research, the persistence of *B. burgdorferi* has not yet been conclusively shown in Lyme disease patients. If it were, it might help explain some of the continuing symptoms that some patients experience following antibiotic therapy.

Future Outlook

Since its initial discovery over forty years ago, Lyme disease has continued to be a growing public health problem in the United States. The recent revision by the CDC of the number of people who are believed to be afflicted with Lyme disease every year clearly shows the extent to which Lyme disease has reached near epidemic status in certain parts of this country. This period has also witnessed many controversies and disagreements among various groups that approach diagnosis and treatment differently, but strive for the same end goal: to lessen the suffering of the people afflicted with this illness.

Despite these troubling aspects, however, there is a light at the end of this very dark tunnel. Recent years have witnessed great advances in technology and medicine, which are being translated into the field of Lyme disease research. Be aware that there is a large group of dedicated doctors and scientists whose purpose is to ultimately conquer this illness. Their success is highly dependent on several factors, funding being at the top of the list. An increase in federal funding for Lyme disease research is critical in order to bring new drug trials, develop new diagnostic tests, introduce methods of tick control, and develop a safe and effective vaccine.

Unfortunately, just when more federal funds are needed, there is less and less tax money being devoted to funding critical scientific research. You can help by becoming active in fund-raising, particularly by lobbying politicians to set aside more money for Lyme disease research. Together, you and the scientists can help bring about positive change in the battle with this disease.

Summary

There are currently many ongoing scientific studies whose sole aim is to prevent Lyme disease or limit how severe it can become. Because ticks and *B. burgdorferi* are the main problems with Lyme disease, scientists have looked at ways of possibly getting rid of both. Some studies looked at reducing the number of deer to see if that would also reduce ticks, while others tried to introduce substances that kill ticks to deer-feeding devices, killing the ticks as the deer feed. To get rid of *B. burgdorferi*, scientists have tried vaccinating mice in the wild. All of these studies show promise in that they either lower the number of ticks or the number of infected ticks. Implementing these programs at a community level will show whether these methods can help in lowering the frequency of Lyme disease.

In addition to these ecological prevention methods, scientists continue to try to prevent Lyme disease by making a new vaccine.

Several new approaches are being tried, which include using a modified version of a previous vaccine or using completely different targets than were used before. Another approach uses a vaccine not to *B. burgdorferi* but to the tick itself, which would cause the tick to fall off soon after the bite and prevent the transmission of all pathogens that may be present in the tick.

Other studies are focusing on trying to improve the current tests that are used for diagnosis, which includes developing tests that can identify several pathogens at the same time. Some scientists are using new state-of-the-art methods such as next-generation sequencing or metabolomics to design better, more sensitive and specific tests and find new pathogens before they even appear in people.

A number of studies are trying to see whether *B. burgdorferi* can really persist after treatment with antibiotics. Because this is a huge point of disagreement in the Lyme community, scientists have used many different techniques to study this topic. The most useful tools for studies of *B. burgdorferi* persistence have been animal models, which are animals that are infected with a pathogen in order to study the disease. Scientists have learned a great deal about the damage *B. burgdorferi* can do in the body from studying animal models. Various animal models have also shown that some bacteria may survive antibiotic treatment. Whether such persistent bacteria can be responsible for any continuous symptoms is a major area of active research.

Further Resources

Centers for Disease Control and Prevention

The CDC website provides all the basic facts about Lyme disease and ticks. In addition, it is also very useful if you are looking for information about tick-borne diseases other than Lyme disease.

www.cdc.gov/lyme/index.html

American Lyme Disease Foundation

Here you will find a wealth of information about all aspects of Lyme disease.

www.aldf.com

University of Rhode Island TickEncounter Resource Center

This center gives a lot of great information about ticks, Lyme disease, and other tick-borne illnesses with a specific focus on preventing tick bites. It can help you learn to identify and differentiate ticks.

www.tickencounter.org

WebMD

www.webmd.com

MedicineNet

www.medicinenet.com

Advocacy Groups

Bay Area Lyme Foundation
www.bayarealyme.org

LymeDisease.org
www.lymedisease.org

Global Lyme Alliance
www.globallymealliance.org

Lyme Disease Association
www.lymediseaseassociation.org

International Lyme and Associated Diseases Society (ILADS)
www.ilads.org

Lyme Disease Network
www.lymenet.org

LymeLight Foundation
www.lymelightfoundation.org

APPENDIX B

Bibliography

Aronowitz, R.A. "The Rise and Fall of the Lyme Disease Vaccines: A Cautionary Tale for Risk Interventions in American Medicine and Public Health." *The Milbank Quarterly* 90, no. 2 (2012): 250–77.

Aucott, J.N. "Posttreatment Lyme Disease Syndrome." *Infectious Disease Clinics of North America* 29, no. 2 (2015): 309–23.

Auwaerter, P.G., and M.T. Melia. "Bullying *Borrelia*: When the Culture of Science Is Under Attack." *Transactions of the American Clinical and Climatological Association* 123 (2012): 79–89.

Auwaerter, P.G., J.S. Bakken, R.J. Dattwyler, J.S. Dumler, J.J. Halperin, E. McSweegan, R.B. Nadelman, et al. "Antiscience and Ethical Concerns Associated with Advocacy of Lyme Disease." *The Lancet: Infectious Diseases* 11, no. 9 (2011): 713–19.

Bakken, J.S., and J.S. Dumler. "Human Granulocytic Anaplasmosis." *Infectious Disease Clinics of North America* 29, no. 2 (2015): 341–55.

Barbour, A.G. "Infection Resistance and Tolerance in *Peromyscus* spp., Natural Reservoirs of Microbes That Are Virulent for Humans." *Seminars in Cell & Developmental Biology* 61 (January 2017): 115–22.

Benach, J.L., E.M. Bosler, J.P. Hanrahan, J.L. Coleman, G.S. Habicht, T.F. Bast, D.J. Cameron, et al. "Spirochetes Isolated from the Blood of Two Patients with Lyme Disease." *New England Journal of Medicine* 308, no. 13 (1983): 740–42.

Bogdos, M., S. Giannopoulos, and M. Kosmidou. "The Conflict on Posttreatment Lyme Disease Syndrome: A Clinical Mini Review." *Neuroimmunology and Neuroinflammation* 3, no. 1 (2016): 10–13.

Borchers, A.T., C.L. Keen, A.C. Huntley, and M.E. Gershwin. "Lyme Disease: A Rigorous Review of Diagnostic Criteria and Treatment." *Journal of Autoimmunity* 57 (February 2015): 82–115.

Burgdorfer, W. "Discovery of the Lyme Disease Spirochete and Its Relation to Tick Vectors." *Yale Journal of Biology and Medicine* 57, no. 4 (1984): 515–20.

Burgdorfer, W., A.G. Barbour, S.F. Hayes, J.L. Benach, E. Grunwaldt, and J.P. Davis. "Lyme Disease—A Tick-Borne Spirochetosis?" *Science* 216, no. 4552 (1982): 1,317–19.

Caulfield, A.J., and B.S. Pritt. "Lyme Disease Coinfections in the United States." *Clinics in Laboratory Medicine* 35, no. 4 (2015): 827–46.

Chang, C., and M.E. Gershwin. "Integrative Medicine in Allergy and Immunology." *Clinical Reviews in Allergy & Immunology* 44, no. 3 (2013): 208–28.

Halperin, J.J. "Chronic Lyme Disease: Misconceptions and Challenges for Patient Management." *Infection and Drug Resistance* 8 (May 2015): 119–28.

Hermance, M.E., and S. Thangamani. "Powassan Virus: An Emerging Arbovirus of Public Health Concern in North America." *Vector Borne and Zoonotic Diseases* 17, no. 7 (2017): 453–62.

Hinckley, A.F., N.P. Connally, J.I. Meek, B.J. Johnson, M.M. Kemperman, K.A. Feldman, J.L. White, and P.S. Mead. "Lyme Disease Testing by Large Commercial Laboratories in the United States." *Clinical Infectious Diseases* 59, no. 5 (2014): 676–81.

Hu, L. "Lyme Arthritis." *Infectious Disease Clinics of North America* 19, no. 4 (2005): 947–61.

Johnson, B.J.B. "Laboratory Diagnostic Testing for *Borrelia burgdorferi* Infection." In *Lyme Disease: An Evidence-Based Approach*, edited by J.J. Halperin, 73–88. Wallingford, Oxfordshire, England: Center for Agriculture and Biosciences International.

Johnson, L., S. Wilcox, J. Mankoff, and R.B. Stricker. "Severity of Chronic Lyme Disease Compared to Other Chronic Conditions: A Quality of Life Survey." *PeerJ* 2 (March 2014): e322. https://doi.org/10.7717/peerj.322.

Kalish, R.A., R.F. Kaplan, E. Taylor, L. Jones-Woodward, K. Workman, and A.C. Steere. "Evaluation of Study Patients with Lyme Disease, 10–20-Year Follow-Up." *Journal of Infectious Diseases* 183, no. 3 (2001): 453–60.

Lantos, P. "Chronic Lyme Disease." *Infectious Disease Clinics of North America* 29, no. 2 (2015): 325–40.

Lantos, P.M., E.D. Shapiro, P.G. Auwaerter, P.J. Baker, J.J. Halperin, E. McSweegan, and G.P. Wormser. "Unorthodox Alternative Therapies Marketed to Treat Lyme Disease." *Clinical Infectious Diseases* 60, no. 12 (2015): 1,776–82.

Marques, A.R. "Lyme Neuroborreliosis." *Continuum: Lifelong Learning in Neurology* 21, no. 6 (2015): 1,729–44.

Mead, P.S. "Epidemiology of Lyme Disease." *Infectious Disease Clinics of North America* 29, no. 2 (2015): 187–210.

Moore, A., C. Nelson, C. Molins, P. Mead, and M. Schriefer. "Current Guidelines, Common Clinical Pitfalls, and Future Directions for Laboratory Diagnosis of Lyme Disease, United States." *Emerging Infectious Diseases* 22, no. 7 (2016). https://doi.org/10.3201/eid2207.151694.

Nadelman, R.B. "Erythema Migrans." *Infectious Disease Clinics of North America* 29, no. 2 (2015): 211–39.

Nelson, C.A., S. Saha, K.J. Kugeler, M.J. Delorey, M.B. Shankar, A.F. Hinckley, and P.S. Mead. "Incidence of Clinician-Diagnosed Lyme Disease, United States, 2005–2010." *Emerging Infectious Diseases* 21, no. 9 (2015): 1,625–31.

Pound, J.M., J.A. Miller, J.E. George, D. Fish, J.F. Carroll, T.L. Schulze, T.J. Daniels, R.C. Falco, K.C. Stafford, and T.N. Mather. "The United States Department of Agriculture's Northeast Area-Wide Tick Control Project: Summary and Conclusions." *Vector Borne and Zoonotic Diseases* 9, no. 4 (2009): 439–48.

Radolf, J.D., M.J. Caimano, B. Stevenson, and L.T. Hu. "Of Ticks, Mice, and Men: Understanding the Dual-Host Lifestyle of Lyme Disease Spirochaetes." *Nature Reviews Microbiology* 10, no. 2 (2012): 87–99.

Rebman, A.W., J.N. Aucott, E.R. Weinstein, K.T. Bechtold, K.C. Smith, and L. Leonard. "Living in Limbo: Contested Narratives of Patients with Chronic Symptoms Following Lyme Disease." *Qualitative Health Research* 27, no. 4 (2017): 534–46.

Rebman, A.W., L.A. Crowder, A. Kirkpatrick, and J.N. Aucott. "Characteristics of Seroconversion and Implications for Diagnosis of Post-Treatment Lyme Disease Syndrome: Acute and Convalescent Serology Among a Prospective Cohort of Early Lyme Disease Patients." *Clinical Rheumatology* 34, no. 3 (2015): 585–89.

Richter, L.M., D. Brisson, R. Melo, R.S. Ostfeld, N. Zeidner, and M. Gomes-Solecki. "Reservoir Targeted Vaccine Against *Borrelia burgdorferi:* A New Strategy to Prevent Lyme Disease Transmission." *Journal of Infectious Diseases* 209, no. 12 (2014): 1,972–80.

Robinson, M.L., T. Kobayashi, Y. Higgins, H. Calkins, and M.T. Melia. "Lyme Carditis." *Infectious Disease Clinics of North America* 29, no. 2 (2015): 255–68.

Sanchez, E., E. Vannier, G.P. Wormser, and L.T. Hu. "Diagnosis, Treatment, and Prevention of Lyme Disease, Human Granulocytic Anaplasmosis, and Babesiosis: A Review." *JAMA* 315, no. 16 (2016): 1,767–77.

Schriefer, M.E. "Lyme Disease Diagnosis: Serology." *Clinics in Laboratory Medicine* 35, no. 4 (2015): 797–814.

Steere, A.C., F. Strle, G.P. Wormser, L.T. Hu, J.A. Branda, J.W.R. Hovius, X. Lin, and P.S. Mead. "Lyme Borreliosis." *Nature Reviews Disease Primers* 2 (December 2016). https://doi.org/10.1038/nrdp.2016.90.

Steere, A.C., S.E. Malawista, D.R. Snydman, R.E. Shope, W.A. Andiman, M.R. Ross, and F.M. Steele. "Lyme Arthritis: An Epidemic of Oligoarticular Arthritis in Children and Adults in Three

Connecticut Communities." *Arthritis and Rheumatism* 20, no. 1 (1977): 7–17.

Steere, A.C., S.E. Malawista, J.A. Hardin, S. Ruddy, W. Askenase, and W.A. Andiman. "Erythema Chronicum Migrans and Lyme Arthritis: The Enlarging Clinical Spectrum." *Annals of Internal Medicine* 86, no. 6 (1977): 685–98.

Telford, S.R., III, H.K. Goethert, P.J. Molloy, V.P. Berardi, H.R. Chowdri, J.L. Gugliotta, and T.J. Lepore. "*Borrelia miyamotoi* Disease: Neither Lyme Disease nor Relapsing Fever." *Clinics in Laboratory Medicine* 35, no. 4 (2015): 867–82.

Theel, E.S. "The Past, Present, and (Possible) Future of Serologic Testing for Lyme Disease." *Journal of Clinical Microbiology* 54, no. 5 (2016): 1,191–96.

Infections Transmitted by Other Ticks

As mentioned in Chapter 2, there are several tick species other than the blacklegged tick that can bite people. Although these ticks cannot transmit *B. burgdorferi*, they can transmit a wide variety of other pathogens. Some of these pathogens can cause severe life-threatening diseases. Probably the two most important ticks, other than the two that cause Lyme disease, are the lone star tick and the American dog tick, especially given that the range of these ticks overlaps with blacklegged ticks. The presence of all these different ticks in the same area can cause even more confusion when your doctor needs to make a diagnosis, especially because many of the symptoms of tick-borne diseases tend to be very similar. The following is a description of all the known diseases that ticks other than blacklegged ticks can transmit in the United States. Being aware of all these diseases, where they occur, and what symptoms you may feel can help you understand what other pathogens you may have been exposed to after being bitten by ticks.

Ehrlichiosis

Ehrlichiosis is a disease caused by several species of the bacteria *Ehrlichia*. The majority of ehrlichiosis cases are caused by infections with *Ehrlichia chaffeensis*, which causes a disease called human monocytic ehrlichiosis or HME. Infection with another species, *Ehrlichia ewingii*, causes a disease called, appropriately, *Ehrlichia ewingii* ehrlichiosis. Both *E. chaffeensis* and *E. ewingii* are transmitted by bites from lone star ticks. In 2011, a new type of *Ehrlichia* was discovered in Wisconsin and Minnesota, two states where lone star ticks are rarely found. This agent was called *Ehrlichia muris*-like or EML, and was later found to be transmitted by blacklegged ticks in that area. There are also other *Ehrlichia* species that typically infect animals, but can on rare occasions infect people as well. Regardless of which species of *Ehrlichia* you are infected with, they are all treated as ehrlichiosis. Overall, approximately 1,000 cases of ehrlichiosis are reported in the United States each year.

🅔❗ Alert

The name *Ehrlichia muris*-like was given to the *Ehrlichia* agent found in blacklegged ticks because of its very close genetic similarity to *Ehrlichia muris*, which is a tick-borne pathogen found in Asia and Japan. EML is generally found in less than 3 percent of blacklegged ticks in the north-central United States and cases are not common. Since 2011, only about sixty-seven have been identified.

The majority of ehrlichiosis cases are reported in the south-central United States, with over 30 percent of all cases occurring in just three states: Oklahoma, Missouri, and Arkansas. The majority of the remaining cases are reported in states located along the Atlantic Coast. The infections are typically reported in the summer, when both lone star nymphs and adults come out to feed.

Ehrlichia infects white blood cells. The symptoms of the disease are likely a result of the inflammatory response to the infection rather than direct damage from the bacteria. The signs and symptoms of ehrlichiosis typically begin within one to two weeks after a tick bite and are very broad. They can include fever, headache, chills, cough, muscle pain, fatigue, nausea, vomiting, loss of appetite, and diarrhea. Occasionally, a rash may appear. The rash is more common in children, where it occurs about 60 percent of the time, than in adults, where it appears about 30 percent of the time. Sometimes respiratory symptoms can appear, such as a cough, with these symptoms being more common in adults than children.

 Fact

The type of white blood cells that *E. chaffeensis* infect are called monocytes, hence the name, human monocytic ehrlichiosis. The name is similar to the disease caused by *A. phagocytophilum*: human granulocytic anaplasmosis. Both pathogens infect white blood cells, but the type of cell they infect is different.

If untreated, ehrlichiosis can develop into a severe disease. About one fifth of untreated patients can develop a central nervous system disease, including meningitis or meningoencephalitis. Deaths from ehrlichiosis occur in about 1 to 3 percent of people who have symptoms. However, many people probably have a mild infection or an infection without symptoms, and don't require treatment.

PCR is most frequently used for diagnosis. If you've been diagnosed with ehrlichiosis, you will be treated with doxycycline. Your fever should subside within forty-eight to seventy-two hours after starting the treatment, which is usually recommended for five to seven days, depending on the severity of your symptoms.

Heartland Virus

Heartland virus is a newly discovered tick-borne virus transmitted by the lone star tick. Infection with Heartland virus is very rare. The first cases of human illness occurred in 2009 in Missouri, and between June 2009 and July 2017, just over thirty cases of Heartland virus disease were identified, most of them occurring between May and September. Most patients reported having a tick bite within two weeks of becoming sick. All of these cases were reported in nine states located within the midwestern and southern United States, including North Carolina, Georgia, Tennessee, Kentucky, Indiana, Missouri, Arkansas, Oklahoma, and Kansas. It is not known if the virus can be found in other states, but it is very likely.

One of the reasons the disease may be so rare in humans is that the Heartland virus is also very rare in ticks. In Missouri, one of the states where Heartland virus disease is most frequently identified, only about one in five hundred lone star ticks is infected with the virus. It is not known whether any other species of ticks can be infected with it as well.

Despite being rarely diagnosed, there may be individuals in whom the infection doesn't show any symptoms or results in a mild, undiagnosed illness. In the patients where the infection was confirmed, Heartland virus caused a severe, life-threatening disease. The initial symptoms of Heartland virus disease include fever, fatigue, decreased appetite, headache, nausea, diarrhea, and muscle or joint aches. The majority of patients diagnosed with the virus were hospitalized, and three of them died. As is the case with the majority of viral infections, there are no medications that can be used to treat the infection. Instead, patients are treated to lessen their symptoms, which includes receiving intravenous fluids and treatment for pain, fever, and any other potential problems.

🔔 Alert

A very similar virus to the Heartland virus is found in China, Japan, and Korea. This virus is called severe fever with thrombocytopenia syndrome virus (SFTSV) and is responsible for thousands of cases of disease each year. The mortality rate of this virus is very high, in some cases approaching nearly a third of infected people.

Currently, diagnostic testing for Heartland virus can be done only in specialized laboratories, and standard testing is not available to the public. If you are suspected of having Heartland virus disease, your samples will typically be forwarded to your state health department or the CDC, where testing for Heartland virus can be done.

STARI
(Southern Tick-Associated Rash Illness)

Bites of lone star ticks will occasionally result in the appearance of a rash at the site of the tick bite that is very similar to the EM rash of Lyme disease. This rash and the symptoms associated with it are called southern tick-associated rash illness, or STARI. Its similarity to the EM rash is so convincing that many doctors are not able to distinguish between the two. Because of this similarity, many people mistakenly believed that lone star ticks could also transmit *B. burgdorferi* and cause Lyme disease. STARI can sometimes be accompanied by other symptoms that appear during Lyme disease, including fatigue, headache, fever, and muscle pains.

However, STARI is not Lyme disease and has not been associated with any other symptoms of Lyme disease such as arthritis, neurological disease, or heart disease. Both the rash and other symptoms disappear after antibiotic treatment with doxycycline. However, it is not known whether the treatment helps to cure the infection or whether the illness goes away on its own. At one time, a new species of *Borrelia* found in lone star ticks, called *Borrelia lonestari*, was proposed to be the agent that caused STARI. However, studies since then haven't found any evidence linking *B. lonestari* to STARI, and the direct cause of STARI is still unknown.

STARI was originally identified in the South, which is how it got its name. However, it may occur throughout the entire range of lone star ticks, including areas where Lyme disease is common. For example, STARI has occasionally been diagnosed in the Northeast.

Because lone star ticks and blacklegged ticks are both abundant throughout the eastern United States, it appears likely that some cases that are diagnosed as Lyme disease are actually STARI.

Rocky Mountain Spotted Fever

Rocky Mountain spotted fever (RMSF) is a disease caused by an infection with a bacterium called *Rickettsia rickettsii*. Despite what you would expect from the name, the disease has a wide geographic distribution, far beyond just the Rocky Mountains, and is present in North America, Central America, and portions of South America. In the United States, *R. rickettsii* is transmitted by three different ticks. The most common tick to deliver the disease is the American dog tick (*Dermacentor variabilis*), which is found throughout the eastern part of the country and along the Pacific Coast. In the West, it is transmitted by the Rocky Mountain wood tick (*Dermacentor andersoni*), and in the southwestern part of the country, by the brown dog tick (*Rhipicephalus sanguineus*). Because the range of these ticks overlaps, RMSF occurs throughout the continental United States. However, it is most commonly reported in the southeastern states, mainly North Carolina, Tennessee, Missouri, Arkansas, and Oklahoma.

RMSF is part of a large group of diseases called "spotted fevers," which are caused by several different species of *Rickettsia*. Spotted fever gets its name from the appearance of a very characteristic dot-like rash that occurs in people with the disease. The rash is a result of the bacteria infecting the cells that line your blood vessels. When they are infected, the blood vessels become less rigid and allow blood to leak out, resulting in the spotted rash. It can appear all over the body but usually begins on your wrists and ankles and then spreads out in both directions. It can move up your arms and legs to your chest and abdomen, and down into the palms of your hands and the soles of your feet. In some cases, the rash may give the appearance of tiny red pin dots, while in others, the appearance of the rash is splotchier. The appearance of the rash may also change the longer you have the disease.

If you have been bitten by a tick infected with *R. rickettsii*, the initial symptoms of RMSF will usually appear about five to ten days after the bite. The first symptoms are a fever and a headache, with the rash developing about two to four days later. Other symptoms you may experience include nausea, vomiting, muscle pains, stomach pains, and loss of appetite. Although the rash appears in about nine out of ten patients, only about half will have it when they first begin to show symptoms. If the rash doesn't appear, the nonspecific symptoms of RMSF can lead to the disease being misdiagnosed. In addition, the small group of patients in which the rash doesn't occur are also in danger of going untreated.

🅔❗ Alert

Along with the three spotted fever diseases, there is also another rickettsial disease present in the United States called rickettsialpox. This disease is caused by *Rickettsia akari*, but is transmitted by mites, not ticks. In most cases, infection with *R. akari* results in a mild illness.

RMSF is a very serious disease that, if left untreated, can progress to severe stages where more than a quarter of the cases result in death. The severe symptoms include encephalitis and meningitis. This may also result in the patient having seizures, experiencing confusion, and being delirious. Some patients can develop shock, which is a critical condition characterized by a sudden drop in blood pressure. Because of the loss of fluid due to damaged blood vessels, some people with the disease may suffer permanent damage to their toes, fingers, arms, and legs, which may need to be amputated, even with treatment. They may also face hearing loss, paralysis, or mental disability. The bleeding that may also occur can damage vital organs, leading to lung, heart, or kidney failure. Most deaths from RMSF occur within the first eight days of the illness. All RMSF infections are effectively treated with doxycycline, which has led to the mortality rate decreasing from about a quarter of all patients fifty years ago to less than 5 percent now.

In addition to RMSF, at least two other tick-borne diseases are caused by other *Rickettsia* species in the United States. One is called *Rickettsia parkeri* rickettsiosis and is transmitted by the Gulf Coast tick (*Amblyomma maculatum*). This disease typically occurs in the Southeast. The other disease is called Pacific Coast tick fever. It is caused by *Rickettsia philipii* and is transmitted by the Pacific Coast tick (*Dermacentor occidentalis* tick). This illness is found in California. Both diseases have similar signs and symptoms, including fever, headache, and rash, but are usually less severe than RMSF. Each year, about 2,000 or so spotted fever infections are reported in the United States. The majority are believed to be RMSF but it is very difficult to tell them apart. Serologic tests for spotted fevers are not very sensitive or specific. They may indicate that you have a *Rickettsia* infection but cannot identify which species. They are also subjective and may cross-react with other agents. PCR is an effective method of diagnosis early in the disease.

Tick-Borne Relapsing Fever

Tick-borne relapsing fever is transmitted through bites of infected soft ticks. The disease is predominantly found in the western part of the country. It has been reported in fifteen states: Arizona, California, Colorado, Idaho, Kansas, Montana, Nevada, New Mexico, Ohio, Oklahoma, Oregon, Texas, Utah, Washington, and Wyoming.

Relapsing fever is characterized by a recurring fever, in which each episode lasts about three days. Episodes are separated by periods of about a week without a fever. In more than half of the patients, additional symptoms appear, including headache, muscle aches, chills, nausea, joint pain, and vomiting. The fever can be very high, up to 106.7°F. Some patients with relapsing fever become delirious and agitated during the fever stage. When the fever drops, you may experience profuse sweating. This cycle can repeat several times if you are not treated. When treated with antibiotics, the symptoms go away after a few days.

Tularemia

Tularemia is caused by an infection with a bacterium called *Francisella tularensis*. It can be transmitted to people by the American dog tick, the wood tick, and the lone star tick. The disease can occur throughout the continental United States. On average, about 125 cases of tularemia occur in the United States annually, with the vast majority occurring in the central and western United States.

Unlike other tick-borne agents described in this book, ticks are not the only vectors of *F. tularensis*. In the western part of the United States, this bacteria can also be transmitted by the bites of deer flies. Other ways that people get infected is by coming in contact with carcasses of animals that died of tularemia. Some people have gotten infected during landscaping by running over dead animals with machinery such as lawnmowers and then inhaling the bacteria. You can also get infected by drinking unclean water or eating food that has the bacteria in it. Very few ticks are typically infected, which contributes to the relatively low number of cases. If tularemia is acquired through a tick bite, it usually causes an ulcer at the site of the bite within the first week, followed by a high fever, chills, headache, diarrhea, muscle aches, and swollen lymph nodes. If not treated, the disease can progress to severe illness and you may die, but the treatment is a quick course of antibiotics.

Colorado Tick Fever

Colorado tick fever is an infection caused by a virus called the Colorado tick fever virus that is transmitted by the Rocky Mountain wood tick. Despite its suggestive name, the disease does not occur only in Colorado but is found in several Rocky Mountain states at elevations of 4,000 to 10,500 feet, which is where the Rocky Mountain wood tick lives. It is also found in Canada.

Most cases of Colorado tick fever occur in the spring or summer. The disease is rare; between 2002 and 2012, only eighty-three cases were reported to the CDC. If you have symptoms, they will begin between one and fourteen days after the tick bite. The most common symptoms are fever, chills, headache, body aches, and fatigue. Occasionally, some patients also report having a sore throat, vomiting, abdominal pain, skin rash, or a stiff neck. About half of all people with Colorado tick fever have two attacks of fever. The first will last several days, go away for less than a week, and then be followed by another fever that will last a few days. In most people, the disease is mild and they will recover completely.

Bourbon Virus

Bourbon virus is another recently discovered tick-borne virus. The virus was first identified in 2014 in a man from Bourbon County, Kansas, who later died of the illness. Only a few cases of Bourbon virus have been reported since then. The symptoms in these individuals included fever, tiredness, rash, headache, other body aches, nausea, and vomiting. Because the virus is so rare, very little is currently known about the disease associated with it. It is currently not clear exactly which ticks transmit this virus, although there is evidence that the lone star tick may be one of them. It is also not clear in what areas of the United States the virus may exist.

Lyme Disease Timeline

1883: First Description of a Lyme Disease Patient

Alfred Buchwald, a German physician, reports the first description of a Lyme disease patient. Buchwald describes a skin disease that has been present in this patient for sixteen years. He calls this skin disease *acrodermatitis chronica atrophicans*, which is now recognized as part of late Lyme disease in Europe.

1909: First Description of the Lyme Disease Rash

Swedish physician Arvid Afzelius first describes a rash that he calls *erythema chronicum migrans*. He also notes that the appearance of this rash occurs after a tick bite. To acknowledge his early contributions, in the 1980s, one of the species of Lyme disease-causing *Borrelia*, *Borrelia afzelii*, is named in his honor.

1920s–1940s: Link Established Between EM Rash and Neurologic Disease in Europe

Various reports from throughout Europe describe the appearance of the rash and a wide range of symptoms of neurologic disease.

1948: First Description of Spirochete-Like Bacteria in Skin Biopsies from Patients with EM Rashes

Dr. Carl Lennhoff suggests that spirochetes may be the cause of the EM rash. Unfortunately, his findings could not be reproduced and were not followed up.

1951: First Effective Antibiotic Treatment of EM Rash

The use of penicillin was shown to be effective in patients with EM rash in Europe.

1970: First Reported Case of EM Rash in the United States

The rash occurs in a patient from Wisconsin.

1975: Alert over the Outbreak of Arthritis in a Connecticut Community

Health authorities are notified of an outbreak of arthritis in and around the town of Old Lyme, Connecticut. These alerts lead to the establishment of a surveillance program in Old Lyme and two of the surrounding towns, Lyme and East Haddam, in order to study the illness.

1975–1976: First Examination of Patients with Lyme Disease

Researchers from the Yale School of Medicine, led by Dr. Allen Steere and Dr. Stephen Malawista, examine groups of patients from Old Lyme, Lyme, and East Haddam who are suffering from recurrent arthritis.

1977: First Characterization of Lyme Disease

Dr. Allen Steere and Dr. Stephen Malawista publish a landmark paper that describes a mysterious outbreak of arthritis in and around Lyme, Connecticut. The disease is initially called Lyme arthritis and is the first definitive study of Lyme disease. A possible link is also made between the appearance of an EM rash and the disease. The authors publish a follow-up study later in the year describing additional patients from 1976. A clear link between the EM rash and Lyme arthritis is made, and ticks are proposed as a possible vector of the disease. For the first time, neurological and heart-related symptoms are linked to this disease.

1979: Geographical Distribution of Lyme Disease in the United States Is Identified

The disease is shown to occur in three areas of the United States: the Northeast, the upper-central region, and the West Coast. It is also noted that the first two areas correlate with the distribution of Ixodes scapularis (then called Ixodes dammini) and the last with Ixodes pacificus ticks.

1980: Antibiotics Shown to Be Effective on the EM Rash

Treatment with penicillin or tetracycline antibiotics is shown to resolve the EM rash in Lyme disease patients and prevent further symptoms.

1982: Identification of the Cause of Lyme Disease

A group of scientists led by Dr. Willy Burgdorfer collect blacklegged ticks on Shelter Island, New York, cut them open in the laboratory, and use a microscope to observe unique, spiral-shaped bacteria inside the majority of the ticks. Analysis of the blood of Lyme disease patients reveals that at some point in the past, all of the patients with Lyme disease were infected with this bacteria.

1982: *B. burgdorferi* Cultured in the Laboratory

The first strain, called B31, is obtained from ticks on Shelter Island and grown in a culture away from any host. The identification of the nutrient mix needed to culture the bacteria greatly simplifies the laboratory study of this organism.

1982: Informal Surveillance of Lyme Disease Begins

The CDC begins to track cases of Lyme disease, but it is not yet a mandatory notifiable disease.

1983: Confirmation of Spirochetes as the Cause of Lyme Disease

The same spirochetes identified by Dr. Burgdorfer are now shown to be present in the blood, skin, and spinal fluid of patients with active Lyme disease, confirming that these bacteria were in fact the cause of the illness.

1984: Lyme Disease Spirochete Is Named *Borrelia burgdorferi*

The bacteria, which up until now were simply called "Lyme disease spirochetes," are named *Borrelia burgdorferi* in honor of Dr. Willy Burgdorfer, who first discovered them in blacklegged ticks two years earlier.

1991: Lyme Disease Becomes a Nationally Notifiable Disease by the CDC

All cases are now required to be reported to the CDC.

1995: Recommended Guidelines Set for Lyme Disease Testing

The two-tiered method using an ELISA and a Western blot test becomes the recommended diagnostic test for Lyme disease, a role it still holds over twenty years later.

1997: Genome of *B. burgdorferi* Is Sequenced

All the genes present in the strain B31 of *B. burgdorferi* are identified, ushering in a new era for Lyme disease genetic research.

1999: Introduction of the Lyme Disease Vaccine

A vaccine called LYMErix, based on the OspA protein of *B. burgdorferi*, is introduced on the market in December by the SmithKline Beecham company.

2000: Lawsuit Is Filed Against SmithKline Beecham and Their Lyme Disease Vaccine

This lawsuit, filed on behalf of vaccinated patients, claims that the OspA vaccine is harmful.

2002: Lyme Disease Vaccine Is Taken Off the Market

Claiming poor sales, the LYMErix vaccine is withdrawn from the market.

2012: Evidence of Persistent *B. burgdorferi* in Monkeys

A study that investigates whether *B. burgdorferi* can remain after antibiotic treatment shows that some bacteria may occasionally be found.

2014: First Study Revising Estimates of Annual Lyme Disease Cases

A CDC study looking at Lyme disease testing by large commercial laboratories in the United States estimates that approximately 240,000 to 440,000 cases of Lyme disease occurred in the United States in 2008.

2015: Annual Lyme Disease Cases Estimated to Be More Than 300,000 per Year

Another CDC study looks at nationwide health insurance claims from patients with Lyme disease and estimates that over 300,000 cases are occurring each year.

Glossary

Antibiotic

A drug used to treat bacterial infections. Most come from natural sources, usually a fungus or bacteria, and are made up of a substance that can prevent the growth of other microbes.

Antibodies

Proteins that help our immune system recognize and destroy foreign microbes. They are somewhat specific to each pathogen, meaning the antibodies that your body makes to fight off the influenza virus will be different than antibodies for *B. burgdorferi*.

Antigenic variation

The ability of a pathogen to fool the immune system by continuously changing the way it looks.

Arthropod

An invertebrate animal with an exoskeleton, segmented body, and paired jointed appendages. Common examples include ticks, insects, and spiders.

Aseptic

Free of bacteria.

Autoimmune response

When your immune system attacks your body's healthy cells and tissue instead of a pathogen. This can cause continuous inflammation, leading to damage inside of your body and persistent illness.

Bacteria

Living single-celled organisms that have cell walls but no organelles or an organized nucleus. The number of species of bacteria are literally incalculable, but there are more bacterial cells than any other cells on this planet.

Bactericidal antibiotic

An antibiotic that kills the bacteria it's targeting.

Bacteriostatic antibiotic

An antibiotic that stops the bacteria it's targeting from multiplying, letting the immune system destroy the bacteria.

Broad-spectrum antibiotic

An antibiotic that can be used against a wide range of bacteria.

Chronic Lyme disease

A disease characterized by persistent symptoms after the treatment for Lyme disease has ended. This illness may include a wide variety of alleged symptoms, such as nonspecific pain, constant fatigue, and various neurocognitive problems and is believed to be, in part, caused by an active infection of *B. burgdorferi*. There is a great deal of debate within the Lyme disease community about whether or not this really occurs.

Cross-reactivity

A test incorrectly detecting one type of infectious agent when it is testing for a different agent. This can cause false positive results.

Culture

Microorganisms grown in a laboratory for scientific studies or tests.

Dead-end host

A host that cannot pass an infectious agent to another person or animal.

DNA sequencing

Determining the order of the four building blocks, called nucleotides, in a strand of DNA. DNA serves as a blueprint of how to make a cell, and determining how it is composed provides a great deal of information about how this cell lives.

Early disseminated stage

The second stage of Lyme disease. At this point, the bacteria has moved through the skin, entered the bloodstream, and spread away from the initial infection site.

Early localized stage

The first stage of Lyme disease. It is characterized by the appearance of a rash at the site of the tick bite as well as flu-like symptoms.

Ectoparasite

An organism that lives outside of a host and benefits from it while causing the host harm.

ELISA test

The first half of the two-tiered Lyme disease test. During the ELISA test, scientists test part of the blood sample for antibodies fighting against the targeted infectious agent. See: Serologic test.

Endemic

A disease often found in a particular area or among a specific group of people. For example, a state with a high rate of Lyme disease is known as a Lyme disease–endemic state.

Erythema migrans

The rash that is the most common sign of Lyme disease. This rash appears at the site of the bite and can vary in appearance.

Hypostome

The feeding tube of a tick. It has serrated edges, giving it a saw-like appearance.

Infection

The invasion of a body by a foreign microorganism.

Infectious agent

Any organism that causes an infection.

Late Lyme disease stage

The third and final stage of Lyme disease. This typically occurs months after the initial infection and is characterized by persistent attacks of arthritis. If untreated, these attacks can continue for weeks, months, or even years.

Lyme-literate doctor

A physician who claims to be an expert at diagnosing and treating patients with chronic Lyme disease.

Microbiome

The collection of every microorganism in an area. That area can be specific, such as your intestines, or broad, such as your entire body.

Molecular test

A test that looks for the physical presence of a pathogen. It increases the amount of DNA of the pathogen that is present in a sample in order for it to be more easily detected. It is also known as a polymerase chain reaction, or PCR, test.

Narrow-spectrum antibiotic

An antibiotic that is specific to a group of bacteria.

Nonendemic

A disease not often found in a particular area or among a specific group of people. For example, a state with a low rate of Lyme disease is known as a non-endemic state.

Pathogen

A microbe that causes disease. Examples include viruses, bacteria, and fungi.

Polymerase chain reaction (PCR) test

See: Molecular test.

Posttreatment Lyme Disease Syndrome (PTLDS)

A condition where persistent symptoms continue after the end of a treatment for Lyme disease. Symptoms can vary, but may include fatigue, joint pain, and muscle aches. Unlike chronic Lyme disease, it is not believed to be caused by an active infection.

Range

The total geographical area where something is found.

Reportable disease

A disease that doctors are required to inform the CDC about when they diagnose a case. This allows the CDC to track statistics and outbreaks.

Reservoir

Any animal that acts as a continuous source of infection.

Sensitivity

The ability of a test to detect a pathogen even if it's present only in very small amounts.

Septic

Infected with bacteria.

Serologic test
A test that searches for the presence of antibodies made to fight against a disease. The one currently used for Lyme disease is known as the two-tiered test, which is made up of the ELISA and Western blot tests.

Sign
A characteristic that a doctor can observe or measure. For example, a runny nose is a sign of a cold.

Specificity
The ability of a test to detect only the specific pathogen that is being tested for.

Spirochete
A type of bacteria that is spiral shaped. *B. burgdorferi* is a spirochete.

Strains
Different types of a specific species of bacteria that contain small genetic differences that can affect how pathogenic they are.

Symptom
A characteristic that you feel but that is not observable. For example, fatigue is a symptom of a cold.

Syndrome
A collection of signs and symptoms that tend to occur together during a particular disease.

Two-tiered test

The ELISA test and Western blot test. Running both together helps clarify any equivocal results and reduce the potential for a false positive. See: Serologic test.

Vaccine

A substance designed to trick your immune system into reacting as if you are infected with a pathogen. This causes your immune system to create antibodies and "remember" the pathogen so if you're ever infected with it in the future, your immune system knows how to react.

Vector

A living organism that can transmit infectious diseases between animals and humans. Examples include mosquitoes, ticks, and fleas.

Virus

The only infectious agent that is not made up of a cell and therefore may not be considered alive. Viruses require living cells to survive.

Western blot test

The second half of the two-tiered Lyme disease test. This test looks for the presence of antibodies for specific proteins. It can also help scientists tell what stage Lyme disease is in. See: Serologic test.

Zoonotic disease

Any disease that is spread between animals and people.

INDEX